NO SIDE EFFECTS
The Return to Herbal Medicine

LaDean Griffin

DEDICATION

To all the silent heroes we call
librarians who catalog and preserve
with a quiet devotion, the writings
of the past, and especially to
Librarian Gary Gillum
of Brigham Young University
for his bibliography of rare books
and to my daughter Lynn
for her help with research.

PREFACE

Have you had the experience of contention with a person who has difficulty drawing his own conclusions, who argues a controversial subject he secretly wants to believe? He demands a logical step-by-step proof by someone he feels is in the know. He invariably attacks this person, by taking the opposite view. He often says, "I don't believe that," so as to draw from his opponent a more convincing argument. After all his questions have been answered in a logical, believable way and with strong conviction, he simply walks away or backs down without saying, "That's right, you are right," thereby leaving a shattering effect on the person so attacked.

If health is what you want, we must learn never to be baited into such a trap. No matter how right or righteous the issues may be, we open the door way for the adversary to enter our lives when we argue.

Those who choose to learn or to gain a testimony by argument are unhappy people. They do not have the ability to way things accurately for themselves, or they are too lazy to dig it out alone. They want someone else to do most of the work and then prove it to them. Because they cause a spirit of contention wherever they go in their quest for knowledge, they become lonely and unwanted. Often they pride themselves on stimulating others to think, at the expense of causing a stir. They commend themselves also on straightening someone out if they happened to find someone who really did not know. In reality, however, he is unsure of himself and is filled with insecurity and personality complexes. Their limited understanding is proven by their neutral and colorless logic, about which Dante commented, *"Let us think no more about them but look once and pass on."*

Much of the quest for truth lies in the spiritual realm we call revelation. In order to maintain health we must learn to avoid argument from either position. Arguments settle in our own brain, after having originated by weeding through books sorting and sifting, on our knees in prayer, and in classrooms where questions are asked but no attacks made. These are the arguments which motivate us, after the contest is over, to sincerely strengthen a conviction which brings inner peace, knowing we have come to our conclusions quietly, alone with God, and have hurt no one in the process. Paul said, *"Prove all things and hold fast to that which is good."*

To learn with the tongue is weakness. To quietly seek after that which is good, proving all things to one's self, is strength and power. Gregor Mendel, Austrian botanist, said in 1882: *"To know what to ask is already to know half."* When one already knows half, it seems inconsistent to let someone else do the rest. The brain is such a marvelous instrument, much like mirrors placed on opposite walls that reflect into infinity. It can think about itself as it thinks about itself thinking about itself.

Those with little knowledge on a subject will often allow themselves to be sucked into argument, soon losing their own way to independent thought. If arguments are continued, they somehow lose the thread of the real story; the issues become disconnected and out of focus. These become the wishy-washy types who after a while are not thinking for themselves.

When we are sure of our own thoughts and convinced beyond doubt it will no longer be important to convince anyone else. Nor will it be important if anyone disagrees with us.

This is where I stand regarding herbal medicine. If you wish to walk with me a while and reason as we go, I welcome your pleasant company. Sincere interest does not entail any risk or complication. It is the beginning of the learning process, the child of wisdom.

The Author

FORWARD

Most of us have observed the effect of a sneeze from black pepper, and crying from peeling an onion. Some of us have felt the effects of poison oak or stinging nettle. Few of us have failed to comprehend the impact of the marijuana plant on our young people. Many of us have recognized that the opiates are in constant use for relief of pain. We all know the effects of tobacco on the body or the effects of certain plants relative to hay fever and asthma. We also seem to know that some plants, such as Hemlock, will kill us; yet there are few of us who know that herbs are an important part of many drug formulas, ointments and medicines, both as an integral part of, or as the beginning of a synthetic drug.

A clever intrigue clearly exists, the well disguised, to wipe from our memories the fact that herbs have any value at all. In many countries of the world, except the United States, the herb Doctor is still looked upon with respect. As the chemical world of drugs was emerged into Vogue any research of the type we know today was drastically limited to drugs and chemicals, leaving the study of plants entirely to the botanist. Much has been done by way of identification – photography, geographical location, etc. yet excludes any useful purpose as far as medicine was concerned.

Meanwhile, the herbalist, who understands the medicinal value in herbs, has been all but forced to silence by the powers that be, branded as a quack, an unreliable idiot hardly worthy of mention. Through these years of indoctrination, the herbalist has managed to survive despite the limitations imposed upon him. Though prohibited from usefully serving mankind with his knowledge, he has continued with dedication to contribute his time spreading the word, so that truth may not be entirely lost during this medical "dark age." Young drug users who finally saw the light, along with the high cost of medical help, have encouraged many people to begin to use herbs, and they have been amazed with the results. They begin to feel as if a whole new world of wonderful, useful, inexpensive knowledge had suddenly burst in upon their brains. All this has given rise to a medical revolution which is gradually becoming a transfer of recognized, established power from expensive hospital and Doctor bills, over to the open field and the herbs that grow about the garden and on the roadsides. If we can keep the leeches from capitalizing on this new market, there could be inexpensive medicine for all.

If we could encourage a systematic search into old herbal methods, and a research into other species of the plant kingdom, we would develop the wisdom to discern that which is intellectual rot from that which is sound knowledge. We may be on the verge of the most wondrous adventure man has yet pioneered.

We may be just a step from the top of the mountain overlooking the Valley where we can get a full, glorious view of all the beautiful plants and trees God has designed for the health and welfare of mankind.

We may find that we have a far grander, more valuable resource than petroleum, potash, gold or silver in health and strength for all.

The author

CONTENTS

CHAPTER 1

ENTER YE AT THE STRAIT GATE

While in a University library searching through some medical books dating back as far as the 15th century, I realized that their value was far greater than simply being of great age. When we see the facts about medicinal herbs which have been so cleverly erased from our generation, we realize that these books resurrect for us some truths that must no longer remain silent. Despite man's ability to land on the moon and his many scientific discoveries during the past 60 years, he has failed to comprehend the wonders of the human body and the plant life around him. Subsequently he has managed to remain only barely alive. He has allowed what was profitable to be praiseworthy and has silenced the lonely voices of protest at their source, observing with approval the physical degradation of men who for all their weaknesses yet have the ability to walk on the moon.

Just as morality is a relative philosophy designed comfortably for the generation in which it resides, so also is health, as when modern man looks upon the average blood count and mistakenly decides that the white count is a necessity. He calls the average sickly man healthy, and knows not what real health and vitality is all about. We will not achieve anything resembling health for another hundred years – if we last that long – unless we change our present course

Who is without pain in our generation? Who is without many moments of depression? Who is without nervousness? As I look at these old books, one singular similarity was always evident as a part of each book. Each author mentions the attempts to hinder the truth he was presenting, the general chaos of a world which too often failed to respond to the knowledge she was trying to teach. He is usually adamant in stating his own defense, which implied, "It's true and I do not care whether you believe it or not!"

In my preface I find myself doing precisely the same thing. As I viewed each book and the writer's knowledge of the herbs, I found myself, as I touched the old pages, being carried back into his world feeling with him the impossible blindness and darkness of the world, and at times the hopeless frustration which attends possession of a truth. My mind could sense that I knew what he knew to be true, and this Scripture crossed through my reflections:

> *"Enter ye in at the Strait gate: for wide is the gate, and broad is the way, that lead us to destruction, and many there be which go in there at.*
> *"Because Strait is the gate, and narrow is the way, which leadeth unto life, and few there be that find it."*

Always in these old writings I felt the thread of hope that must attend the physician who has confidence in his remedies. Still I could feel his grief for those who failed to obey the rules or whose bodies were too far gone for any remedy to help. Holding these old books in my hands, I felt the infinite power that transfers light and knowledge from heaven source, into the corruptible, breakable, weak, pitiable, but glorious, tangible mind of a man, and can relay it on to subsequent generations of other men who seek truth even against raging tyranny.

As I thought about these learned scholars, my mind reflected over the situation today where people who preach natural methods are expected to live forever, and when they become sick or die, their method is blamed. The fact that in many cases they did not begin a health program until long after a life filled with broken rules and dissipation, was not noted or considered at all.

A Doctor in the medical field, on the other hand, can lean over our bed, red puffy-faced and drippy nosed and we somehow expect nothing of him as far as his own health is concerned. We seek no example of him. If his patient dies observing established rules of treatment, no one is blamed, no one really cares but the loved ones. These comparisons alone should imply something. Somehow, more is expected of the preacher of natural methods. It is as if we all secretly know within our being, regardless of the propaganda or lethargy that surrounds us, that nature is all wise and truly the great healer. It could be compared to the smoker – drinker who turns to his non-smoking friend and says "You don't have any bad habits," or the fact that we seem to instinctively know cake or candy is bad for us. We somehow know that when much truth is given much is expected.

Only when we are free from the burden of hunger do we have time to find understanding and gain an additional knowledge. Only then does man have time to create beauty, culture, music and art. America has had this freedom from want. Now has been the time to search for more positive spiritual and physical answers, but we have been lost in the maze of chemical therapy. Individualism and specialism has been intensified to an almost primitive ritual, selfishly disregarding the group or what is good for the world environment in general.

Have we really gone too far down the wrong road? Have we broken too many universal laws for so long that we must be forced back to the struggle for existence so as to bring us to that reality which brings things into a better focus, preparatory to flowering forth again to correct development? Yes, for unfortunately we have created a growing cultural heritage of immorality inconsistent with the God fearing strength that built this nation.

Evil, greed, and wealth under such circumstances become a burden as the righteous obstinately resist until they gradually adjust themselves, and religion sanctions evil, and a nation deteriorates into chaos.

Do we have to accept gracefully the evil designs of wicked men in the last days, or can we live above the storm? Can we think for ourselves, pray, and find comfort, solace, and strength without being ashamed or worrying about being singled out as a peculiar people?

With human effort and righteous obedience can we have the faith to expect and receive supernatural aid? James Gibby said:

> *"Many of us live far below the character standards we are capable of achieving, simply because we fear the criticism or crave the approval of those among whom we work and live. But never allow such lack of approval to keep you from high resolve or noble deed, for even a fool does not respect a fool."*

Must we live with the wicked who steal from the weak, cheat the stupid and sanctimoniously are fairly honest with the rest? Must we become essentially akin to degenerate men who daily lives between treachery and robbery in commerce and trade? Or can there be a refinement of life profoundly perceiving that which is clean-cut and right rather than that which is only barely distinct between right and wrong?

Any time in history when great men have, through the depths of their souls, then touched with the light of heaven, their progenitors receive this spark of deity in a timeless, classic writing which somewhere deep in the human soul rings a bell of remembrance of a good world, of the past when we lived with a loving Father in Heaven. Those sensitive souls who have been sickened by man's inhumanity to man in their day to day world, as well as in history, find a moment of peace, knowing someone else has received intense spiritual power and adorns the world with a reflection of sweetness and goodness somewhere, sometime, somehow, amid the squalor of this repelling environment, so that they, because of these classics can begin to build their own pillar of faith with gratitude.

Somehow these moments shared with genius have an electrifying effect on those tender souls who are concerned about the sins of the world. The majority, however, though touched momentarily, refused to allow it to fill them further, so they apathetically walk away from the spark which could be a beginning to problem solutions. It is the few who find a way and see the light who helped to maintain the old writings, the old paintings, the old wisdom, and who agree that our ancestors were not all ignorant barbarians. Rather, there have been those sensitive, loving, few all down through time, who by their literary and artistic forms created an ennobling shrine from which we can gratefully draw strength and hope for the future.

This is how I felt as I caressed these old pages, knowing what I do about herbs and their influence as food and medicine. I was lifted in confidence and justified in my own understanding. I could feel the immense role that these great men of the past with dignity and grace, under tyranny and oppression, felt impelled to write, and speak out anyway, that they may pass it on to those few successors who were seekers of truth.

As I give the lists in this book, herbs for symptoms, I will list the names of the early doctors who use the herbs, and will give any biographical information which I might have available.

Chemicals

Living in a chemical world as we do, degenerative disease and hospitals are excepted parts of our existence. Are such diseases really an essential part of aging or merely that which we have come to expect? In certain remote areas of the world, such as in Hunza land, people live to useful old age while retaining their faculties up to ages of 100 years or more.

We add such chemicals as benzoic acid, dimethyl polysiloxane DDT, parathion (a potent phosphorous nerve gas pesticide) and saccharine to the fruit and fruit juice we use. Then we add the pesticides chlorine-dioxide to our flour, and methoxychlor, chlordane, heptachlor, toxaphene lindane, DDT, benzene, herachloride, aldrin, dieldrin, and stilbestrol (artificial sex hormone) to our meat. To our potatoes we add pesticides and sulfuric preservatives. To peas we add magnesium chloride (to retain color) magnesium carbonate (to alkalize), DDT parathion, methorchlor, malathion. To our salad vegetables with dressings, we add sodium alginate (as a stabilizer) monoisopropyl citrate (as an antioxidant preventing fat deterioration) DDT, phosphorus, insecticides, and weed killers.

To our bread we add ammonium chloride (dough conditioner) Mono and diglycerides, polyoxithlene (softness),diterthiary-butyl-panacresol (antioxidant), nitrated flour or coal tar dye (to give a yellow color suggestive of eggs or butter), vitamin fortified DDT and parathion.

To our butter we add nondihydro-guaiaretic acid (antioxidant), magnesium oxide (neutralizer) AB or OB yellow coal tar dyes, and diacetyl (artificial aromatic agent) DDT.

To pickles, aluminum sulfate (to firm), sodium nitrate (to give texture) and emulsifiers are added.

To ice cream carboxymethyl cellulose (stabilizer) Mono diglycerides (emulsifier) artificial color and flavor, coal tar dyes, antibiotics DDT are added.

Along with the well-rounded diet, we are accumulating all these toxic substances. As I have mentioned in my book *Is Any Sick Among You?*, a person with an inadequate hormone balance cannot even handle the so-called well-rounded diet. What do they think we could do with all these added toxic substances, when most of what would normally sustain life already becomes toxic in their bodies? People say to me quite often, "I live on a good diet. I take vitamins and herbs. Why is it I am still unable to cure this disease or improve any further than I have?" Until we stop this senseless intake of poisons and chemicals, we will always be sweeping more trash in the front door than we can sweep out the back, so, on we continue into degenerative disease and old age. There is all the difference in the world between farm people who live out in the sun, raise their food and their own un-poisoned meat and milk, to people living in the crowded, bizarre vibrations of the city, working indoors all day and living on devitalized, man poisoned, factory prepared, foodless foods.

There should be some way to put a stop to these evil and designing men who make a living from devastation of the public health. You may say, "we have the FDA to protect us." How many chemicals enter the market daily until the FDA can catch up with them? How many singularly not very toxic chemicals do we eat in a day found in first one food and then another? How many of these accumulated chemicals does it take to be toxically poisoned? Yes, we all want help, and long life, and freedom from pain. But if we are to achieve these far-fetched dreams, we must pay the price and grow much of what we eat or somehow rid ourselves of the evils of chemicals from our society.

Herbs are not as pleasant a replacement for nutrients as those found in fruits and vegetables, grains, etc. and were not intended to replace more palatable food. Their function is to regulate organs and glands, correct the balance, and cleanse the cells. Over a century ago Americans started the most costly experiment in history – living on refined foods and at the same time discontinuing the general use of herbs, using synthetic drugs for medicine instead. This has proven to be a disaster to the general health of the nation.

Most American housewives know nothing about the wonderful aromatic gourmet use of condiment herbs which enhance, not only flavor, but increase the ability of the body to use and digest the food.

Ellen G. white wrote nearly a century ago:

"God has caused to grow out of the ground her herbs for the use of man, and if we understand the nature of these roots and herbs, and made right use of them, people would be in much better health than they are today. These old-fashioned, simple herbs used intelligently would have recovered many sick, who have died under drug medication."

Drugs

"With all his conscience and one eye askew, so false he partly takes himself for true."

Rudyard Kipling

With a new sense of collective purpose, the world is taking a more critical look at medical sciences basic assumptions, high medical costs and the possibilities of sustained health. More and more people have come to realize that drugs cause a chain reaction in the body as explosive to well-being as an atomic bomb. The main support of drug research has come about because of the wealth of the nation, it's irrational hope that some magic pill could restore health and somehow bypassed the laws of nature and the inevitable punishment for his departure from obedience to those laws which govern his body. Most often he becomes sincerely disturbed by anyone who tries to inform him what that law is.

Shakespeare said:
"I find the medicine worse than the malady."

This has become far more true in our own time that during the time of Shakespeare.

In a recent newspaper, the experts blame an estimated 140,000 American deaths annually, caused needlessly by adverse reaction to drugs. It was noted that an estimated cost to the American people for these adverse drug reactions was $2 billion per year. It was also noted from studies of hospitals throughout the nation that 30% of hospitalized patients, or about 8.7 million, have drug reaction, and 14% of all hospital days are devoted to care of patients with a drug reaction. Of all hospital admissions 3 to 5 percent are for drug reaction. It was also noted from researchers' studies that 8 common drugs produced one third of all adverse drug reaction. The most dangerous problem came from the interaction of combining certain drugs.

The blame for these alarming figures was, of course, given to the physician who did not look into a patient's past history or did not know enough about the drugs in question: How can a patient give an account of the drugs he has taken when the prescription is kept so secret from him? How can he even get the information from his past physician when such professional jealousy exists? Then, lastly, how could most doctors keep up with John Doe if they would pass on his past record while he runs the gauntlet from one doctor to another because he becomes worse and worse as he endlessly seeks the answer to his problem?

In my possession is a Physicians Desk Manual which lists all prescription drugs on the market. If you were to read it from cover to cover, it would be the most frightening thing you could ever read. Were you to understand from the physician's own book just how adversely these drugs could act in your body, you would, I am sure, never take another drug. We have all been partly responsible as we have helped to establish the medical power in this country as we place the physician in a godlike position with all-knowing power. The ads pour forth from the communications media, "Be sure to see your doctor."

How people can be afraid to use the time proven herbs that are listed as far back as recorded history, is beyond my ability to comprehend, when they are always used for the same purpose and yet have no fear of being subjected to the trial and error chemical therapy which is ever-changing.

In my own life time I remember the splash ads in the newspaper about the wonder drugs during the war. Then I recall the quiet notices as discoveries were made about the damage they had done. We have all seen this time and again. How long will we deny the gift of the spirit by trusting in the arm of flesh? We have allowed science to contaminate our food, our water, our air, and our bodies with inorganic poison. How long will we continue to raise the proud banner and boast of man's great medical attainments? With the pollutants we receive and absorb into our bodies, an attempt to gain spiritual energy is an almost feeble, insignificant gesture.

How can we study history objectively and continue to be led down the Primrose path to destruction by unscrupulous men who have built powerful drug companies to get gain from the unsuspecting, duped, uninformed public, all in the name of the progress of man? It may require increasingly higher prices on food and products, higher living, insurance and medical costs to remove man from the insanity of drugs. We may then discover to our amazement, how our grandparents survived without running to the doctor for every little ache or pain.

My paternal grandmother always gathered, dried, and used herbs with great knowledge, while my maternal grandmother was never without certain herbs on her pantry shelf.

II Timothy 3:7 states that man is:

> *"Ever learning, and never able to come to the knowledge of the truth."*

Is it possible, medical science has been but a Fata Morgana (mirage) that we have been hoodwinked into believing by a propaganda method well known to all of us?

Before we are all wasted by "evil designs of wicked men in the last days," perhaps now is the time to at least establish enough contempt for half-truth and falsehood so that we may by degrees, rid ourselves of dangerous, indifference to truth.

History is often shown that it takes war, famine or pestilence when a nation is close to the brink of dangerous weakness, before the prophets will again be heeded and its people whipped out of the worshiping of individualism and egomania.

For a time, man then regards the group with respect, the prophets with honor, and his fellowmen with unselfishness, learning to share instead of reaching endlessly for his neighbor's purse.

Within the pages of the old books I have listed, there is always an undercurrent of spirituality by those writers who had a correct understanding of bodily functions. My impression has been that a true scientist never allows the spiritual man within him to die no matter how much pain he may achieve in his clinical skill. Somehow, all truly great physicians, feel the weakness and solitude that accompany the heavy burden of the life and death situation which confronts them. Because of this feeling, they seem to know their own ability. Knowledge does not always suffice, so they cannot afford to be cut off from the sustaining contact with the Infinite Intelligence which could give revealed answers to their problems.

It has also been my observation that wherever specialization has advanced, the physician becomes more impersonally detached toward his patients, losing somewhere along the way the need for close contact with God. Perhaps his road is too well-traveled and narrow rather than widespread and vast. He seems to feel secure in his own knowledge and needs no help from the Infinite. He may become a leading academic figure but that touch of sensitivity which reaches out from him to touch those intimate cords of human feeling, which bring peace and comfort to his patient, is lost by his Scholastic self-assurance.

In reading these old books, I find the thread of obnoxious abominations being used with such great confidence and an all-knowing attitude that repeatedly these remedies have had a favorable reaction on their patients. As I noted the use of such ingredients as crushed crab eyes added to the apothecary or the powdered skull of a man, I recalled the words of Oliver Wendell Holmes:

> *"Whatever elements nature does not introduce into vegetables, the natural food of all animal life, directly of herbivorous, indirectly of carnivorous animals – are to be regarded with suspicion. The disgrace of medicine has been a colossal system of self-deception, in obedience to which mines have been emptied of their cantankerous minerals, the vegetable kingdom robbed of its noxious gross, the entrails of animals taxed for their impurities, the poison bags of reptiles drained of their venom, and all the inconceivable abominations thus obtained, thrust down the throats of human beings suffering from some fault of organization, nourishment of vital stimulation."*

An example of obnoxious abominations being used with such confidence:

Joannes Groenevelt (1649) in *A Treatise on the Safe Internal Use of Cantharides* dedicated his book to Lord William Earl of Portland, gentlemen of the bedchamber to his late Majesty King William.

On pages 16 – 17, he talks about a Spanish fly or beetle used to make a medicine which has a diuretic effect. He says Avicen said little could be done without cantharides.

He quotes Hoffman:

"that they could not by other means provoke urine"

On pages 70 – 73 he said that Oil of Camphir kills and expels worms. It expels stones and is good for uterine ulcers, gout, fever, plague and spotted fever.

As I reflected on these things that may seem to the sophisticated, modern man, an obnoxious stupidity used by an ignorant barbarian of the past, I wondered just how far we have come when we use the pus from cow pox or the urine of a pregnant woman (the latest fad for losing weight to the tune of $25 a shot, while she still goes on a 700 calorie a day diet)? Just how far have we really come when we still seek, as have the ancients, to find purity and immaculate health from the abominable things which nature tries to discard as waste. The interesting thing in this new urine fad is that it is being used to counteract or stop the process of elimination. Where it is shown on the blood test as a high toxic condition and heavy mucus elimination, it has been found that the taking of urine shots stops the mucus.

Still man stumbles along, not recognizing how the body feeds and eliminates and that elimination of mucus waste is nature's way to save life. The doctors of the past seem to recognize that they must purge the body in order for it to recover, but here and there they seem to have missed the point when they added some obnoxious, abominable thing which caused a jolt, forcing the body to do something in the same manner that drugs react. When man finally learns that drugs and this sort of thing merely stimulate the body to further elimination to get rid of the drug being administered (but in the final analysis only weakens and destroys) he will begin to approach the light of the true knowledge that could bring him to immaculate, beautiful health.

Somewhere, somehow, if man is to survive and be well, he must learn what manner of fuel is correct in order to be rewarded with such health. If man is to create a more spiritual world, where peace and love can exist, he must cease filling his body with such abominations that rot and putrefy the body as well as the drugs and alcohol that destroy his reason and judgment.

How can he expect to be loving, kind and tender when his body is racked with pain and filled with filthiness?

How can he expect to tap the spiritual realm of existence with all the corrosion on his physical wires?

The time may come when we will recognize that our bodies have more to do with electrical power, and that our spiritual power makes a better contact with cleanliness than with filth. The time may come again as was in ancient Israel that ill health will be looked upon with contempt as a sin, and the question will be asked "What have you been eating?"

This may be the reason Christ said, as he healed the sick:

"Thy sins be forgiven thee."

CHAPTER 2

HEALING NATURALLY

John Douglas (1665 – 1743), Manuscript, Lessons on Surgery, page 38, says:

When any man discovers a new and useful operation or makes any advantageous improvement of an old one, he's been sure to be persecuted as a bold innovator by the bulk of his own fraternity.

The following information I give as my opinion on subjects not covered in my book *Is Any Sick Among You?*

Rheumatoid Arthritis

My opinion about Rheumatoid Arthritis is that it is a disease of the peripheral joints, and the early signs are usually fatigue, weight loss, muscular aches, stiffness in the joints, pain, a feeling of warmth in certain areas, and usually swelling. It comes on in acute stages of severe pain, swelling, and inflammation. It is a disease not understood by modern medical science because it falls into the category of an acute condition similar to a cold. Since a cold is not understood, the treatment of this painful type of arthritis has been merely to suppress the pain by the use of aspirin. When using heavy doses of aspirin, often the patient is much distressed by an upset stomach. No matter what other medications are used, the basic aspirin regimen is usually continued.

We have not come very far from the old alchemists in their use of metal compounds when we use gold injections to suppress Rheumatoid Arthritis. Patients who have taken gold eventually suffer far more than the immediate pain of arthritis. Since these metals are not assimilatable into the body, a continual buildup and develop into a more serious disease.

It has been found that the anti-malarial compounds modify this type of arthritis. This brings me to the conclusion that there are certain parasites involved, possibly the tubercular Bacillus, or the malarial parasite. The malarial parasite can be killed by the use of Black Walnut powder. The tubercular Bacillus can also be killed by Black Walnut.

There is a tie-in between Rheumatoid Arthritis and the disease Lupus. Lupus, being a disease of the connective tissues, is caused by the tubercular Bacillus. Both of these diseases are caused in the beginning by adrenaline malfunction. As the body builds and accumulates toxic waste from the lack of its ability to throw off the waste, in a weakened condition caused by hormone imbalance, parasites readily find food to propagate their young. As these parasites increase in number, the mucus they live upon is retained in the body. Even on a cleansing, semi-fasting or fasting diet, they seem to be able to hold onto their food supply. Therefore, it is important to kill the parasite so that the mucus they live on will be set free to eliminate. Since parasites are the cause of the bodies inability to throw out the mucus, even when mucus is acutely gathered in the bloodstream, it merely circulates from one place to another. Wherever it is more solidly accumulated at a given time, pain is manifest; however the entirety of the body remains in an acute condition, leaving the person tired and sufficiently weak to desire to remain in bed. Most often however, people with this disease will keep going regardless of the pain or the fatigue.

The adrenocorticosteroids-related cortisone compounds have been used with some success for this type of arthritis because it has usually been brought about by adrenaline exhaustion where the cortin hormone has not been produced. When cortisone was discovered it was found to be helpful for this type of arthritis. Rheumatoid Arthritis is not a gradually degenerative disease but rather a sudden manifestation as a result of a traumatic experience: death in the family, shock, accident, overstressed in business or family. A complete exhaustion of the adrenal glands is caused due to overproduction hormone necessary to handle the stress.

Steroid therapy with the use of cortisone could have been an important advance in medical science had they not determined to manufacture the hormone synthetically. There have been many disastrous side effects from the use of cortisone, and people with all types of arthritis where the adrenal gland is not the cause, have demanded this drug, causing more complications, until the medical doctors have become discouraged with the drug. It has been used in many cases of skin condition, caused by the same adrenal malfunction, where if the person did not break out and release the toxic waste, they would be in serious pain from arthritis. Man often brings about a worse condition by attempting to stop natures illuminative processes.

To use natures remedies would seem far more reasonable. The herbs that acts like steroid cortisone is licorice root. The synthetic drug has been made from Mexican wild yam. It would seem that the logical method to follow would be: cleansing the waste from the body, increasing the body's ability to use food, correcting the chemical balance by adding the licorice, this would allow the body to act as if it had created the hormone, thus increasing its ability to utilize starches and meats until such time as it may produce on its own these necessary hormones, then by killing the parasites feeding upon the accumulated toxic mucus, a healing crisis would slough off the mucus. It has been my experience to watch the wonders of a healing crisis when parasites have been killed. Globs of mucus will pour forth from the body. (See "Healing Crisis" in my book, *Is Any Sick Among You?*)

Lupus

Systemic lupus is a disease of the connective tissues. The skin seems to be affected in a similar way to a person with Addison's disease, where freckles or patchy blotches appear on the skin –

usually unexposed areas of the body. It has been found under close medical supervision that the malarial drug is beneficial but does not solve the problem. There seems to be a connection between the adrenals and this disease. A cortisone compound has been used with some success, but for the most part, the disease is considered terminal.

It is my opinion that Rheumatoid Arthritis and Lupus may be closely related. If the tubercular bacillus which they are trying to put to sleep with the antimalarial drug could be killed and cleansed out of the body, than a correct intake of better, less-toxic foods would gradually rebuild the deterioration of connective tissues. When the connective tissues of the body are hanging like a rag, causing the bones to rub and touch rather than be cushioned, there can be pain similar to that of arthritis. The connective tissues in Lupus is more widely extended throughout the entire body. When analyzing the eyes, as in Iridology (from the Iris of the eye), Lupus is seen by white lines appearing between the color lines wherever the acute degeneration is occurring. In Rheumatoid Arthritis the eye will appear very white over the color of the iris itself. This white will be widespread and more intense wherever inflammation occurs. There also appears the white line of the Lupus between the color when the superficial white does not completely cover it from view. In some cases, there may be brown spots specifying the joint areas of the iris, which indicates a disease of long-standing and degeneration of the bones. Degenerative arthritis, on the other hand will usually appear only as brown chronic spots in the bone structure segment of the Iris.

Since it is known (as in the science of iridology) that white indicates healing or an acute condition on the move out of the body, as with a cold, leukemia, or any virus disease, it should logically follow that Lupus, as well as Rheumatoid Arthritis, should be a condition easily moved. In most cases however, this is not the case. The waste simply stirs around in the bloodstream, unable to be removed from the body. This brings me to my conclusion that parasites are involved. The body's ability to throw off waste is retarded and weekend by a constant accumulation of parasites. When the parasites are killed, nature has a better chance to cleanse and rebuild.

Medical science notes an extreme anemia. Corticosteroids are used in treatment because of adrenal involvement. Such cases usually have a history of pleurisy.

A brief home remedy is listed below:
Restorative doses $B_2 - B_1 - B_6$
Black Walnut or full parasite formula
Licorice approximately 2 to 4 caps a day
Folic acid
Multiple vitamin
Vitamin E
High doses of vitamin C

Arthritis Osteoarthritis (Degenerative)

Gradual changes in cartilage and joints, particularly in the spinal area, are characteristics of this type of arthritis. The assumption is that constant wear and tear has caused the breakdown in degeneration. Only a small percentage of people with this type of arthritis have any distressing symptoms. A shearing away of cartilage occurs leaving bone against bone. It is also a wasting or wearing away of the bone itself. The most common symptom would be stiffness and aching pain, worse after much activity. The pain can be disabling and constant, especially if it is in the knees or hips. Overweight and lack of muscle tone creates added burdens on the joints. A skeleton may be stood up by holding it by the head, but if you drop it, it falls in a heap. It takes muscles to hold bones in place. And strong muscle tone takes the burden off the joints. To say that we must lose weight, stay off the joints, rest, exercise, or take pain pills would be treating the effect and not removing the cause requires high potassium to maintain strength of muscle tone. Calcium, phosphorus, and vitamin D are required to prevent the deterioration of the bones. In addition, a sound hormone balance is needed to utilize the foods properly so as to prevent a toxic buildup.

The thing suggested by today's method of treatment would be like driving your car without tires. When stress is a cause factor, overcoming stress by resting is often an impossibility. We sometimes have a tiger by the tail and cannot let go. It would be better to have a natural hormone which would act as if the body had produced it. Sufficient nutrition then rebuilds the body so that one could stand whatever stresses life had to offer.

When men have lived to such great age in the past it does not seem reasonable to me that deterioration by 50 years old should become, as it has in our society, an accepted hazard. We in the United States, during the past 50 years, have become a degenerate people both physically and spiritually. How can we expect to stand up to the stresses of life? We must learn to eat the foods necessary to well-being. In the beginning to bring about health changes, a mild food diet, vitamins and herbs, is recommended as outlined in my book, *Is Any Sick Among You?*

For my purpose in this book I will only list the herbs useful to the treatment of general arthritis. There may be a time when we are unable to obtain natural vitamin products, so it is important to understand which herbs of the field are helpful in specific cases of disease.

With tongue-in-cheek, some testing has been done in certain hospitals recently on the use of chaparral for arthritis and cancer. Where only tea and incorrect diet were used, there was, of course, a non-predictable result followed by an attitude of, "We knew that was of no value, just a psychological, all-in-their-head, sort of thing when people have gotten better." It has been proven to me and to many others repeatedly during the past 25 years that teas are a very weak substitute for whole or powdered herbs. Sometimes to become accustomed to certain herbs, teas are useful as a start or where fasting is involved. For use with babies, they are excellent, but for chronic disease in adults they are ineffective. There is a lot of talk about tinctures and certain oils being brought out of the plants by cooking. It is my personal opinion that only in emergency, as with seizure or with evacuation of the stomach, are they superior to live, uncooked herbs. Dividing and separating each attribute, as the young alchemists are learning to do with herbs, only continues the mistakes we have already made with drugs. An individual factor will merely act as a drug to shock or jolt the body into some action. My feeling is that we should be tender and careful, even in the process of elimination. Take it easy and slow; nature's way is not a sudden and immediate, but a gradual healing process. We live in such a world of "instant this" and "instant that" we somehow expect to take a pill for instant health. The interesting thing about herbs is that they can be used alone, or dozens of them may be used together without the side effects caused by mixing drugs or alcohol. Often a better result is achieved by using many herbs that complement each other.

Nature is still, in the final analysis, kinder than we suppose. It will not take as many years to overcome the disease as it took to arrive at such a state of degeneration.

Listed are the herbs helpful for general arthritis:
Alfalfa
Black Walnut (for parasites)
Celery
Chaparral
Licorice
Mandrake (as laxative)
Nettle
Peppermint
Pumpkin Seeds (for parasites)
Solomon's Seal
Wild Yam
Wood Betony

It seems appropriate to me at this time, to point out that ossification is the normal deposit of calcium in the tissues and bones, whereas calcification is the excessive deposit for infiltration of calcium into sick, dying, or dead tissue, as a result of the reduction of the body's ability to throw off waste. Excessive deposits are often caused by too much uric acid in the blood, which holds the calcium in deposit in the joints. Certain herbs, such as celery, alfalfa, chaparral, and saffron, have a tendency to return this calcium into solution and move it on out. They appear either to have the ability to neutralize these acids or regulate the hormone balance. Whichever it is, it works. Calcification and infiltration are proof to me that the body has not been receiving sufficient calcium, potassium, magnesium, phosphorus, and vitamin D for its use in maintaining sufficient tone to prevent calcification. Certain cases of osteoporosis occur when the bones become hollow and insufficient. At times this hollowing is caused by the tubercular bacillus, and we call it bone cancer. We may again draw a relationship. Nevertheless, there is not enough material to maintain the bone structure being utilized by the body. This again brings us to the conclusion that we may need herbs to kill the parasites, and foods and herbs to rebuild a finer, more solid structure.

The facts about parasites are hideous but inescapable and problems with them will continue to persist until we learn how to keep our bodies clean and free of the mucus and wastes upon which they feed.

Gout

Gout is a degenerative disease also, where there is a defect in the body chemistry, leading to an accumulation of uric acid. The urate crystals deposit in the cartilage, causing a sudden acute attack manifested by an inflammation of the joint usually at the base of the big toe. Pain or swelling can be present anywhere in the leg. It might be interesting for you to know that certain drugs, including aspirin, can elevate blood uric acid even though they are used to suppress the pain. People with gout usually will develop kidney stones later on from too much uric acid. The normal treatment on examination would be to draw the fluid from the inflamed joint or to use aspirin and a drug known as colchicine, which is made synthetically from meadow saffron. It has a remarkable effect, somehow being able either to dissolve or to increase the ability of the patient to use oil, which is generally the cause of uric acid buildup. It is interesting that some people who lack sufficient adrenal hormone production when on a reducing diet have too much fat moving into the bloodstream from their own body fat this will build uric acid, causing an acid burning in the stomach and in the entire body, with the possibility of later developing kidney stones. It is been my experience that since the herb, saffron works, it would be better than the synthetic drug in assisting the body's ability to use oil. In cases where the glands are not producing adequately, such things as fried foods, potato chips, etc., are unable to be digested. The use of saffron allows digestion of such negative foods. It is not that I believe that we should use the antidotes for disobedience to the law; however, it may help to know the answer when we have offended nature. In the case of any degenerative disease, the rule is always mild foods, vitamins, and essential herbs. When the body has a defect in chemistry, leading to an accumulation of any waste product, the answer is always to cleanse the system. When the body is cleansed, pain and inflammation are removed, because where chronic disease is concerned, pain is only a manifestation of accumulated waste.

Cancer

In my book *Is Any Sick Among You?*, I give some excellent cancer formulas, but I do not discuss cancer to any great degree. In writing again a little more on the subject, I wish to state again my Constitutional right of free press as a citizen of the United States to say what I believe to be true. There have been many brave souls in the past whose exuberant worship of reason and justice have been brought quickly down to paralyzing disillusionment and they have found themselves shorn of any consoling faith in their fellow men because they dared to tell a truth about herbs. Bacon said:

"History is the planks of a shipwreck. More of the past is lost that has been saved."

As we look back into history and try to reconstruct the bits and pieces of true medical knowledge, we discovered that the world is and always has been filled with darkness, and only a few here and there really tried to find out or cared to know at all. We console ourselves with the thought that in order to remain sane, most people try to forget many of the bad experiences they have had, so they stumble and make the same mistakes time and again. If we could learn to dismember these bad experiences of pain and sickness for neat handling long enough to think through just what we did and just what we ate at the time, we may be at the beginning of analytical wisdom. We may also have arrived at the place where repentance could make a substantial impact on our lives.

William Beckett (1712), in a letter to a friend, *New Discoveries Relating to the Cure of Cancer*, made the observation that Quicksilver will dissolve gold, aqua fortis (iron), vinegar

(eggshell), and oil (sulfur). Why not something to dissolve hardened tumors?

He talked about not being slaves to the opinion of the ancients (page 15):

"No, this would be to strangle truth, and extinguish the vigiorus of our wits with precarious authorities."

He related cures by certain famous physicians: Monsieur Alliot, position to Duke of Lorrain; Doctor Hoberfield, principal physician of Bohemia; Sleur Gendrom, Doctor of physick, University of Montpelier.

On page 24 he said the application of dissolvent to breast cancer brought off a quarter of a pound of it in 3 to 4 days and took 3 months to dissolve it all. He used a tincture of Myrrh for final washing and finish.

Beckett tells about his new discoveries relating to the cure of cancers, wherein he rejects the painful method of cutting them out or off, but rather recommends dissolving the cancerous substance. He gives instances of his success in such practice on persons reputed to be incurable.

On page 30 he said that cutting was not often attended with success.

He speaks on page 36 of surgeons becoming sick from the cancer juices touched in the patient.

Although cancer has not been considered a communicable disease, there may be some basis in fact concerning what William Beckett says about the juices of a sick cancer. If another person were in a ready condition, with fertile ground for bacteria to grow, the disease could be as contagious as tuberculosis. There has been a great deal of research done, and many effective methods, not accepted by the United States medical profession, exist with which the cancer can be killed. It is well and good to kill the cancer, but it is also necessary to be able to get it out of the body before parasites move-in and take up new residence in the remaining cancer. The cancer may also be obstructing vital organs of the body. It would make more sense to help it to Slough off into the blood and be gradually eliminated from the body.

This is exactly what these herbal cancer formulas, along with a mild food diet, are able to accomplish. After a few months, the body may have a healing crisis and force any cancer or tumor out of the body at the nearest bodily opening: the bowel, vagina, lung, or throat.

Where cancer is far extended in the body, the destruction of the cancer is dependent upon body vitality or the ability and strength to throw it out. Also, when the formula may not be in sufficient strength to kill extensive cancer, chaparral in strong amounts up to 8 - "00" capsules a day over and above the formula may be added with great help. Sometimes it is necessary also to kill parasites living in the cancer before it will slough off, using in addition pumpkin, black Walnut, and other vermifuge herbs. After the cancer has been killed, it is essential to move it out of the body, and it is important that it not move too fast so as to obstruct or become clogged in the blood or in the bowel. A mild food diet, laxative herbs, such as are found in the cancer formula, and enemas almost daily will be helpful.

George Cheyne (1671-1743) in *The English Malady*, in the preface stated that meat and protein in man, along with spirituous liquors, will make their pains and sufferings less both in life and death.

In Chapter 1, page 7, he notes that the body has lost its ability, tone, elasticity and force in fibers or nerves in particular. He recognizes the body is full of swellings and tumors. Ulcers or hardened glands must be emptied of their waste, but he still sees that to stop the elimination or pain with meats and liquors helps to relieve pain.

In some cases this may be true, as protein stops the elimination process and changes the body from acute pain to chronic disease. In other cases, such as cancer death and many gland or kidney deaths, meat cannot be tolerated or handled at all. It has been known that a cancer case too far gone to heal, where pain is intense, can find relief of pain by use of grape juice only and the person can do without the painkillers and so remain rational until the last.

It was my extreme pleasure to read recently about certain research which claims, as I have always believed, the cancer is filled with parasites. The discovery that has been made is that certain parasites, such as the tubercular Bacillus, make a change in form to what is called the Progenitor Cryptocide. In this same research, they also found parasite involvement in cardiac problems. When we know the cause of all disease, we are immediately aware that this is so.

We understand that disease is caused by an over-encumbrance of waste from incorrect eating habits, wrong combinations of foods, or inorganic, inherent weakness causing any imbalance in the gland and body mechanism. Because of any or all of the above reasons, the body begins its lymphatic retention of waste; when it remains too long and is not forced out by a cold, or moved out by a semi-fasting or fasting condition, the years of accumulation become food for the parasite whose function in all of life is to remove that which is imperfect and return it to dust so that new life may begin again in perfect state.

In the plant kingdom any imperfection or fault in growth causes the bugs to respond to their eternal reason for existence.

Modern man grows faulty plants with chemicals, and when the bugs appear he sprays the plant with poison to kill the bugs, and eats the sickly plant nature would have destroyed. Thus he destroys himself in the process because his poor nourishment invites the internal parasite to bring the faulty mechanism back to dust. Man does the same with his body as the grower when he gives penicillin to kill the parasites and germs rather than to properly feed the body that it may be well.

When we use the parasite herbs and kill the growing death within us, have we solved the problem if we do not rebuild the body to sound resistance? Until we learn to live on organically grown, healthy food and in the correct combinations and amounts, excluding chemicals and drugs from our bodies, we can be nothing but food for the parasite. When we learn that it is not the bacteria nor the parasite that are our enemies, but rather the abomination of drugs, chemicals and chemically grown poor nourishment, we will then be on the road to longevity and real health.

Epilepsy

At times, those in the urban field, become so excited about the use of certain herbs they somehow believe that their pet herb is good for everything. It is important to know enough about pathology to decide whether a disease requires a sedative or stimulant type of herb. Where the nervous system is concerned, stimulants are not to be used, as they excite the nervous system even further. In the case of epilepsy, the sedative drugs are used such as Dilantin, phenobarbital, etc., which keep the patient in an almost drugged, low, quiet state. Epileptic people who have changed over to the nervine type herbs suddenly seemed to come alive. The world takes on a whole new bright awareness. Drugs will often kill the male sperm so that a woman taking them continually is not able to conceive. A story was told to me recently about a boy who had not even been able to control seizures with dilantin and was taken off the drug by an overzealous herb enthusiast, put on high, close doses of cayenne. This caused the boy to go into seizures every 2 minutes. The boy had to be rushed to the hospital and put back on the drug until he quieted down. He was later put on the nervine herbs, high doses of B complex and calcium to feed and quiet the nervous system, along with a mild food diet and has been much better. Others, convinced that drugs were detrimental, have tried these methods and found an amazing, new and wonderful world of health not known before.

As the toxic waste is being moved out of their bodies, the seizures will be further apart but will be more violent. Then they will become less violent and further apart.

When a person is taking Dilantin, phenobarbital, etc., folic acid is destroyed in the body – and folic acid is essential to the use of B_{12}. The glands can then become affected from the lack of B_{12} until they are often unable to produce hydrochloric acid. Menstrual disturbances, vision problems, spinal cord, degeneration, and muscle cramps will follow. These would be considered side effects from drugs because of the destruction of the body's ability to use B_{12}.

Certain types of epilepsy are caused by brain damage. Other types are caused when the axis vertebrae of the neck is out. These cases have been completely cured by putting the vertebrae back into place. Other types are caused from a toxic condition of the colon. When the colon is restored to normal by herbs and mild food the seizures will cease.

Often a convulsion is caused by an obstruction in the bowel. Sometimes fainting and blackouts are the results of the same problem. Because medical science is back in the dark ages when it comes to a knowledge of care of the colon and how the body feeds and eliminates, it is missing much of the cause of an epileptic seizure. It is interesting to read what the doctors of the past new about falling sickness or seizure.

William Salmon (1644-1713), *Doron Medicum:*

His understanding on how to treat the epileptic was shown by the many patients who were cured by purge and physick. It was obvious that he understood quite well that elimination played a great role in overcoming this disease.

Phlegm in the brain is a cause of epilepsy (page 279). Cold feet immediately affect the brain. He also said morning and noon sleep begets catarrh (page 280).

He used hyssop, wormwood, and betony for epilepsy. He gave case histories of bleeding and bloodletting, with good results (page 719).

He gave a formula for epileptic lunacy:
Ginger

Cinnamon
Mace
Clove
Nutmeg
Cubebs
Peony (the root was often used by ancient physicians)

As I read the old books written by William salmon, I am impressed by his power of logic, the depth of his understanding, the widespread scope of his knowledge and his ever-seeking analytical, scientific mind.

The iris of the eye (iridology) will show epilepsy as a brown or white line or spot on the epileptic center of the eye. The medulla area of the brain on the eye will show either brown or white. It is also of interest to note that the autonomic nerve wreath of the eye will show white or brown. (Where only white is showing on all three places, this would indicate no brain damage.)

The colon area of the eye will usually, in this type, be toxic brown in color indicating that the seizures are caused by the toxic colon. There are times when constant seizure, even though caused from the colon, will result in brain damage. Without expert help it is difficult to determine sometimes. The neck area of the eye should be double checked not only for brown spots or white but for nerve rings crossing the spinal area of the eye. This would indicate the cause as the axis vertebrae being out of place.

In all cases, the autonomic nerve wreath of the eye will be affected either showing brown or white: brown being chronic; white being acute

In order for it to be epilepsy, the epileptic center, brain medulla and nerve wreath would all be involved and would show up on the Iris of the eye.

With any of the three reasons I have shown, the mild food diet, nervine herbs, high vitamin B factors, and calcium are a far better answer to epilepsy than drugs.

When the colon is the cause, the CS formula or laxative-type herbs, slippery Elm, and B6 assist the body to clean and clear the colon of the toxic waste causing the problem.

When the neck is the cause, a good chiropractor would be necessary to place the vertebrae in its proper place. When the cause is brain damage, the herbs and diet are still superior to drugs, in order to lessen the seizure problem as well as assist the body in utilizing vitamins and minerals and to remain well in all other respects.

Any time the herb Lobelia is used as a nervine, cayenne should be used in small amounts, but for no other reason should cayenne be used on an epileptic person.

Stroke

In cases of a chronic brain syndrome caused by a stroke or brain damage when there is danger of seizure, the nervine herbs, B factor and calcium for more oxygen to the brain make it possible to keep down the danger of seizure or violence without the use of tranquilizers or harmful drugs. Often in these cases the blood sugar is also low, and licorice root provides help in added resistance to fatigue as well as the necessary hormone lacking. The frustration from not being correctly functional in speech or mobility, etc., can cause a drain on the adrenal stress factors to a point where hypo- or hyper-glycemia becomes a party to the problem.

Here again cayenne should only be used if Lobelia is used. In all nervous problems cayenne is too high a stimulant to be indicated. When the nerve wreath on the eye is either white or brown (acute or chronic) the body is in need of quieting, soothing, healing herbs and vitamins. Even when there is complete nervous exhaustion (breakdown, fatigue) it would seem logical to give cayenne to stimulate, but it is not the correct herb in this case.

Before the nervous system can heal, it must be quieted and rebuilt with corrective food and vitamins. Too often, even in degenerative disease such as cancer, tuberculosis, diabetes, and related gland problems, the nerve wreath shows involvement. Therefore, it is important to quiet and heal the nervous system if the body is to build sufficient vitality ability to throw off the disease. In most gland problems, especially diabetes, the nervous system is deeply involved.

Parkinson's disease

Certain drugs or chemicals administered to normal people can cause all symptoms of Parkinson's disease within 2 weeks.

Since it has been decided that chemical substances can produce these symptoms, it would indicate the immediate cause must be toxic chemicals accumulated in the basal ganglia, slowly causing damage. It is thought also that a faulty liver may contribute to the accumulation.

Medical science is still hoping to find an antidote drug to arrest the progress of the symptoms which are caused by the drugs. Hyoscine, a natural plant product, is used against tremor by medical doctors. B_{12} shots are also used. Dryness of mouth, blurred vision, nausea, constipation, and slow urinary stream are the most common side effects caused by drugs.

Surgery is not looked upon by medical science as a method of solving the problem, because it can cause impaired mental sharpness and speech problems. The thing that is most discouraging to them is that the problem returns after surgery.

Somehow it does not ever occur to medical science that Parkinson's disease could be a degenerative nervous disease caused not only from drugs, which they themselves acknowledge, but from lack of proper nutrition to maintain the body with enough vitality to throw off the drugs.

The fastest and best way to rebuild is raw vegetable juices and mild, mostly raw food. High restorative doses of vitamin and mineral supplements, using especially the high B factors and calcium.

Many of the so-called terminal diseases would be no longer considered terminal if people could only learn how to eat the proper foods and clean their bodies of accumulated toxic waste.

Wilson's disease

Wilson's disease is a rare degenerative disease of the corpus striatum (the tail-like, lens shaped nuclei of the brain) and cirrhosis of the liver, characterized by distortions of the muscles (actively increases distortion), difficulty with speech, stammering, difficulty in articulation of joints, and difficulty in swallowing. It is thought that its cause is faulty copper metabolism.

Yet it has not occurred to medical science that the inability to correctly metabolize copper could be caused from the lack of other related minerals and vitamins in the body. Among natural health circles, it seems a simple thing to use high amounts of vitamin and mineral supplements and lots of fresh, raw vegetable juices, fresh fruit, along with a mild food diet, to normalize this problem. It is caused from eating too many concentrated foods, such as meats, starches, and sugars. When the reverse is practiced, the result is health restored.

All the old writers clearly understood that the cause of disease was toxic waste buildup in the body. The first thing our grandmothers did when someone was sick was to give a laxative, an enema, or both. Herbs have a way of assisting nature in her determined course, that of forcing an elimination of waste to save life and in the process adding necessary nutrition. If we could learn to keep our bodies clean and eat correctly we would have the help we so much desire.

CHAPTER 3

USEFUL HERBS

People ask me all the time, "How do you know how much to take" and "How many herbs can you combine?" The fact is, each herb can be a combination of many healing factors. As you go through the lists you will see some herbs listed many times. These, of course, are the greatest healers. Nature can do many things at a time like the human brain; different properties work together like a fine machine to accomplish many purposes.

You can yourself combine many herbs to make a formula which will achieve even more.

When we understand how the body feeds and eliminates, it is a simple thing to note that herbs cleanse and regulate all systems. With the information that there is only one disease (the retention of waste) and all other illness is caused by an organic fault in the mechanism, it is relatively simple to decide which herbs are needed. When we know what each herb will do, such as increase the flow of urine or act like a hormone we are not producing, etc., we can decide quite simply which herbs we need to add to our diet.

The general rule for making a base formula would be:

Laxative (to cleanse bowels)
Tonic (to tone and restore)
Diuretic (to help kidney elimination)

Nervine (all healing is subject to nerve ability)
Vermifuge (kills parasites)

If the person were slow or sluggish, then a stimulant can be added.

If the person were hyperactive, no stimulant would be indicated.

If the glands were out of balance, then, of course, the hormone herbs should be added.

If other known organs were not functioning correctly, the herbs specific to that need, such as heart herbs, etc., would be needed.

Where vitamin or mineral deficiency is the cause and vitamins and minerals are not available, the herbs will prove most helpful. Alfalfa is one of the best overall (highest in all vitamins and minerals) values known. Lobelia is the fastest general obstruction mover and sedative. Cayenne is the best stimulant. Juniper is the best (kidney) diuretic. Goldenseal Root is the best antibiotic. Slippery Elm is the best to soothe and heal. Black Walnut and pumpkin are the best for parasites. Then if we add the few hormone herbs, it becomes a relatively simple thing to take care of any illness. There is, however, an overwhelming list of useful herbs we could learn about but we can start with only a few.

It is my opinion that for serious disease, teas are not the answer unless raw herbs are used in unheated water. The whole powdered herbs stirred into water or placed in capsules work to the best advantage. However, the teas work very well for babies.

At this point I would like to attempt without sure knowledge, to speculate as to what happens when hard narcotic drugs are used versus the use of herbs. The medical books themselves tell us that medicine and drugs cause more poisoning fatalities than all other combined chemicals and that half of the poisoning deaths in children are caused by aspirin. The barbiturates and hypnotics are the drugs most frequently the cause of adult deaths by poisoning. Then other poisoning deaths commonly reported are caused by antihistamines, laxatives containing strychnine, and analgesics containing opiates. In the modern field of drug medicine, we find any narcotic drug name ends with "ine" as does the word medicine. Words such as morphine, codeine, quinine, heroin (diacetylmorphine), cocaine, dextro-amphetamine (STP), amphetamine (Benzedrine biphatamine), methamphetamine (desoxyn methedrine), mescaline, the belladonna alkaloids (atropine, hyoscine, hyoscyamine) and so on. There seems to be endless number of brand names ending in "ine", but this is a clue to their narcotic addictive effect. Some are made from opium, some from other alkaloids sources such as peyote or cinchona, etc. the full 10% alkaloid substance found in opium, for example, is the part that is used to make heroin-morphine.

It is my speculative opinion that these concentrated opiate alkaloids cause the body to alkalize immediately, somehow resulting in a given psychosis, change in blood pressure, hallucinations, confusion, tremors, slurred speech, lethargy, excitability, restlessness or whatever, depending upon what is used. It seems to me to be possible that these drugs are not directly connected necessarily with the brain to cause such effects, but could rather be an effect upon the entire body, creating an immediate violent change in alkaline-acid balance. It is also my belief that all pain, which is not caused by injury, is the direct result of mucus or acid-bound waste in the body. As the body becomes cleaner and more free of such mucus obstructions, it becomes alkaline. This is the healing process. Man has, however, used with most powerful narcotic herbs and taken the single alkaloid factor to relieve pain by this sudden change.

We know that too much waste on the move in the blood causes acute illness and pain, but when it reaches the delirium stage, the pain is not felt. This is what I believe happens with a concentrated alkaloid, an immediate change over to the point of delirium. Then, as the body changes back to acid, pain begins and with more intensity. In this way, the drug becomes addictive.

With the acid drugs, such as alcohol and L.S.D. etc., I believe the exact opposite occurs, causing a sudden change to an acid condition, similar to a disease crisis, which results in delirium, hallucinations, confusion, etc. Then when the acid is lowered, through evacuation of bowels, through kidneys or eliminated through the skin, the confusion begins to subside. We can see how such violent changes could cause injury or death. In my opinion, the poison and heavy narcotic herbs should not be used even in a natural state, or anything that shocks the body in any way. There may be much more to the alkaline-acid balance than we at this time suppose.

Certainly I do not know all the answers, but I do know that the cleaner and healthier the body becomes the more alkaline it is, and too quick a change back to a concentrated meat and starch diet requiring certain acids for digestion is done with difficulty.

Modern man has tried to outsmart God by his isolation of individual factors and in taking the alkaloid from opium, he has certainly caused more pain in this world than he has relieved. When man learns the cause of disease and changes his eating habits, he will no longer need drugs to relieve pain, except perhaps for injury. When the body is clean, free from waste and well-nourished, it bleeds little, heals rapidly, has no infection, and feels less pain. To live with the mild herbs and food is the route to health, and in this way we can live without the side effects of drugs.

If you can train yourself to learn the properties and usefulness of each of the herbs I have listed, it will be a beginning into a wonderful experience, and you will prove to yourself as you use these herbs and obtain a good result that nature is the great healer.

There are many more to be learned. Listed are only a few by comparison, but I have tried to give the most commonly known so that you can begin from there and go on as far as you can with the knowledge of herbs.

HERBAL FUNCTIONS

ALTERATIVE

Function – Healthful change without having evacuation, gradual change to correct, purify impure blood

Black Cohosh
Blue Flag
Blue Violet
Burdock
Butternut
Celandine
Chickweed
Cleaves
Cornsilk
Daffodil (William Salmon, *Doron Medicum*, 1644 – 1713)
Elder (flour, leaves, bark, root, or berries)
Gentian (William Salmon)
Herbane (William Salmon)
Kelp
Lily (William Salmon)
Maidenhair (William Salmon)
Mallow (William Salmon)
Mandrake
Milkweed
Motherwort (William Salmon)
Plantain
Poke Root
Prickly Ash (bark or berries)
Red Clover
Red Raspberry
Sage (William Salmon)
Sanicle
Sarsaparilla
Sea wrack
Spikenard (William Salmon)
Squaw Vine
Wild Lettuce (William Salmon)
Wild Oregon Grape
Yarrow
Yellow dock

ANADYNE

Function – for relief of pain

Barefoot Root
Bittersweet
Cornsilk
Hops
Lobelia
Motherwort (Joseph Smith, *The Dogmaticus or Family Physician,* 1829*)*
Mullein
Pleurisy Root (Joseph Smith, *The Dogmaticus)*
Poppy (Joseph Smith, *The Dogmaticus)*
Solomon's Seal
Thorn Apple (Joseph Smith, *The Dogmaticus)*
Valerian

ANTHELMINTIC

Function – expels worms

Buckbean
Butternut Bark
Gentian Root
Hops
Hyssop
Pink Root (Benjamin Smith Barton, *Collection for an Easy Materia Medica,* Part I, 1798)
Quassia

ANTIBILIOUS

Function – promotes activity of the bile – nerves, Biliousness

Balmony
Mandrake

ANTIDOTES

Function – against poisons

Bloodwort (Joseph Smith, *The Dogmaticus)*
Onions (Joseph Smith, *The Dogmaticus)*
Plantain (Joseph Smith, *The Dogmaticus)*
Skullcap (Joseph Smith, *The Dogmaticus)*
White Ash (Joseph Smith, *The Dogmaticus)*

ANTIEMETIC

Function – stops vomiting

Colombo
Red Raspberry

ANTISEPTIC

Function – counteracts putrefaction

All Heal
Beech
Bethroot
Black Walnut
Black Willow
Myrrh
Plantain
Violet Leaves and Flowers
Water Pepper
White Oak Bark
Wild Alum Root
Wintergreen
Wormwood

ANTISPASMODIC

Function – relieves or prevents spasms

All Heal
Black Cohosh
Catnip
Cayenne

Seed run
Chamomile
Lady slipper
Lobelia
Mistletoe
Motherwort
Mullein
Pleurisy Root
Rosemary
Rue
Sage
Self-heal
Skullcap
Skunk Cabbage
Spearmint
Thyme
Valerian
Wild Yam

APERIENT

Function – gentle laxative without purge – helpful where there is weakness

Birch Root (Joseph Smith, *The Dogmaticus)*
Bittersweet
Blue Cohosh(Joseph Smith, *The Dogmaticus)*
Boneset (large doses)
Burdock
Cleaves
Dandelion (Joseph Smith, *The Dogmaticus)*
Elder flowers
Periwinkle
Plantain (Joseph Smith, *The Dogmaticus)*
Rhubarb
Saffron (Joseph Smith, *The Dogmaticus)*
Vervain (Joseph Smith, *The Dogmaticus)*

AROMATIC

Function – stimulant; spicy, pungent taste

Anise
Basil
Bay Leaves
Bayberry
Birch
Bungle weed
Burnet Root
Calamus
Chamomile
Caraway
Catnip
Celery
Hyssop
Lavender
Magnolia
Marjoram
Peach
Penny Royal
Peppermint
Rue
Saffron
Sage
Sassafras
Spearmint
Wormwood

ASTRINGENT

Function – contraction and stops elimination; tones and firms tissue, muscles, arteries, skin, loose teeth, etc.

Aloe Vera
Bay Leaves
Bayberry

Black Cohosh
Black Walnut
Black Willow
Bungle weed
Comfrey
Cranes Bill (Joseph Smith, *The Dogmaticus)*
Evening Primrose
Eyebright
Fireweed
Fleabane
Horsetail
Magnolia
Mullein
Nettle
Periwinkle
Peruvian Bark
Pilewort
Plantain
Queen of the Meadow
Red Sage
Redroot
Rhubarb
Sanicle
Skullcap
Self-heal
Shepherd's Seal
Squaw Vine
St. John's wort
Strawberry
Uva Ursi
White Oak Bark
White Pond Lily Root
White Willow
Wild Alum Root
Which Hazel
Yarrow
Yellow Dock

CARDIAC

Function – healing for the heart

Hawthorne Berries

CARMINATIVE

Function – expels gas

Angelica
Anise
Balm
Bay Leaves
Calamus
Caraway
Catnip
Coriander
Cubeb Berries
Dill
Elder Flowers
Fennel
Ginger (Joseph Smith, *The Dogmaticus)*
Masterwort
Mint
Penny Royal
Peppermint
Pleurisy root
Rosemary
Rue
Spearmint
Thyme

CATHARTIC

Function – evacuating to the bowels

Aloes

Barefoot
Bitterroot
Boneset (Joseph Smith, *The Dogmaticus)*
Butternut Bark
Castor Oil (Joseph Smith, *The Dogmaticus)*
Hydrangea
Mandrake
Poke Root
Rhubarb(Joseph Smith, *The Dogmaticus)*
Salts(Joseph Smith, *The Dogmaticus)*
Senna

DEMULCENT

Function – soothing, relieves inflamed areas internal or external

Cornsilk
Flaxseed
Ginseng
Gum Arabic
Lungwort
Marshmallow
Parsley
Peach
Psyllium
Slippery Elm
White Pond Lily Root

DEOBSTRUENT

Function – remove obstructions

Bittersweet
Goldenseal Root
Mandrake
Nutmeg
Plantain
Poke Root
Prickly Ash

White Pond Lily

DEPURATIVE

Function – purifies blood stream

Bittersweet
Dandelion
Red Clover
Sanicle
Yellow Dock

DETERGENT

Function – cleansing to wounds or to boils and piles

Agrimony (Joseph Smith, *The Dogmaticus)*
Bittersweet(Joseph Smith, *The Dogmaticus)*
Black Walnut
Burdock(Joseph Smith, *The Dogmaticus)*
Dandelion
Pile Ward
Psyllium
Red Clover
Sarsaparilla(Joseph Smith, *The Dogmaticus)*
Sassafras(Joseph Smith, *The Dogmaticus)*
Yellow Dock

DIAPHORETIC

Function – increases perspiration

Angelica
Anise
Balm
Birch
Black Cohosh
Boneset (small doses)
Buchu

Catnip
Colts foot
Coral Root
Dill
Elecampane
Fennel
Hyssop
Lobelia
Origanum
Penny Royal
Pleurisy Root
Red Sage
Rosemary
Sassafras
Spikenard
Yarrow

DISCUTIENT

Function – dissolvent of tumors

Chickweed
Elder
Sanicle
White Pond Lily

DIURETIC

Function – increases flow of urine

Apple Tree Bark
Aspen
Balm of Gilead
Bitterroot
Bistort Root
Bloodroot
Buckthorn Root
Burdock
Carrot (Joseph Smith, *The Dogmaticus)*

Celandine
Celery
Chicory
Cleaves
Cubeb Berries
Dandelion
Elder Flowers
Elecampane
Fennel
Fleabane
Fo-ti-tieng
Goldenseal Root
Horehound
Horsetail
Hydrangea
Juniper Berries
Lobelia
Mullein
Nettle
Parsley
Peach
Plantain
Pleurisy Root
Pumpkin Seed (Joseph Smith, *The Dogmaticus)*
Queen of the Meadow
St. John's wort
Palmetto
Sea Wrack
Strawberry
Sumac Berries
Turkey Corn
Twin Leaf
Uva Ursi
Violet
Watermelon (Joseph Smith, *The Dogmaticus)*
White Ash
Wintergreen
Wood Sage
Yarrow

DORIFICKS

Function – sweating

Burdock Seed (Joseph Smith, *The Dogmaticus)*
Catnip (Joseph Smith, *The Dogmaticus)*
Chamomile (Joseph Smith, *The Dogmaticus)*
Marjoram (Joseph Smith, *The Dogmaticus)*
Penny Royal (Joseph Smith, *The Dogmaticus)*
Pleurisy root (Joseph Smith, *The Dogmaticus)*
Saffron (Joseph Smith, *The Dogmaticus)*

EMETIC

Function – produces vomiting

Bearsfoot
Bitterroot
Bittersweet
Blue Violet
Boneset (large doses)
Buckthorn Bark
Celandine (wild)
Elder Berries
Fire weed
Giant Solomon's Seal
Holy Thistle
Lobelia
Mandrake
Mistletoe
Poke Root

EMMENAGOGUE

Function – promotes menstruation

Aloes
Bethroot

Black Cohosh
Blue Cohosh
Marjoram
Mint
Motherwort
Mug wort
Myrrh
That make
Parsley
Penny Royal
Rag wort
Rosemary
Rue
Sumac Berries
Sweet Balm
Tansy
Thyme
Vervain
Water Pepper
Wintergreen

It is interesting that so many condiment household herbs are useful to this problem. Since it is a common complaint, common and easily accessible herbs are provided.

EMOLLIENT

Function – softening, soothing on parts that are inflamed

Elder
Elder Flowers
Slippery Elm

Slippery Elm is one of the most soothing herbs for ulcers, internal or external. It is healing for inflamed colon or bladder.

EXPECTORANT

Function – draws mucus facilitating expectoration

Bloodroot (Joseph Smith, *The Dogmaticus)*
Boneset (small doses)
Coltsfoot
Elecampane
Honey
Hyssop
Lemon
Lobelia (Joseph Smith, *The Dogmaticus)*
Blood wort
Mandrake (Joseph Smith, *The Dogmaticus)*
Myrrh
Nutmeg
Peach
Pleurisy Root
Ragwort
Red root
Sanicle
Seneca (Joseph Smith, *The Dogmaticus)*
Skunk cabbage
Solomon's Seal
Violet Leaves and Flowers
Yerba Santa

FEBRIFUGE

Function – stops or reduces fever

Apple Tree Bark
Aspen
Balm
Blood Root
Coral Root
Hyssop
Magnolia
Parsley
Peruvian Bark
Poplar

HEPATIC

Function – helpful for liver disease

Beet
Dandelion
Lemon
Spearmint

LAXATIVE

Function – increase bowel action

Apple Tree Bark
Barberry
Bearsfoot Root
Black Walnut
Blue Violet
Burdock
Cascara Sagrada
Chicory
Elder (Joseph Smith, *The Dogmaticus)*
Goldenseal Root
Motherwort
Mullein (Joseph Smith, *The Dogmaticus)*
Mustard
Peach
Saffron
Senna
White Ash

MUCILAGINOUS

Function – soothing to inflamed parts

Buckthorn Bark (Joseph Smith, *The Dogmaticus)*
Chickweed
Comfrey (Joseph Smith, *The Dogmaticus)*

Flaxseed
Gum Arabic
Lungwort
Marshmallow
Psyllium Seed
Sassafras (Joseph Smith, *The Dogmaticus)*
Slippery Elma
Solomon's Seal
Wild Turnip (Joseph Smith, *The Dogmaticus)*

NARCOTIC

Function – powerful anodyne hypnotic; relieves pain, produces sleep

Bittersweet
Bungleweed
Wormwood

NERVINE

Function – soothing to nervous system; calming to nervousness

Borage
Catnip
Cedron
Hops
Lady Slipper
Lobelia
Motherwort - 46, 47, 49, 58
Prickly Ash Bark and Berries -
Rosemary
Rue
Sage
Skullcap
Valerian
Vervain
Wood Betony

NUTRITIVE

Function – high mineral and vitamin content

Alfalfa
Birch Bark
Black Willow Bark
Bladder Wrack
Burdock
Burdock Seed
Calamus
Carrageen
Carrot Leaves
Catnip
Cayenne
Chamomile
Chickweed
Cleavers
Coltsfoot
Dandelion
Devils Bit
Dulse
Elderberries
Eyebright
Fennel
Fenugreek
Grape Leaves
Hawthorne Berries
Hops
Horsetail
Iceland Moss
Irish Moss
Kelp
Lamb's Quarters
Licorice
Marigold
Meadowsweet
Mistletoe

Mullein
Nettle
Oak Bark
Okra
Oregano
Paprika
Parsley
Planting
Primrose
Red Clover
Red Raspberry
Rose Hip
Rue
Saffron
Sanicle
Shepherd's Purse
Silver Weed
Skunk Cabbage
Slippery Elm
Sorrel
Strawberry Leaves
Watercress
Waywort
Wintergreen
Yarrow
Yellow Dock

PARASITICIDE

Function – kills parasites

Black Walnut
Pumpkin Seeds

PURGATIVE

Function – produces copious discharge from the bowels

Celandine

Violet (William Salmon, *Doron Medicus,* 1644 - 1713)

REFRIGERANT

Function – cools the body

Barberry
Chickweed
Cleaves
Sorrel
Sumac Berries

RESOLVENT

Function – dissolves tumors and pus

Elder Berries

SEDATIVE

Function – tonic for nerves; quieting

Bungle weed
Cleaves
Evening Primrose
Peach
Saw Palmetto

STIMULANT

Function – increases functional activity, nervous sensibility, promotes body energy

Anise
Aspen
Bayberry
Bearsfoot Root
Black Cohosh (Joseph Smith, *The Dogmaticus)*
Burdock

Cayenne (Joseph Smith, *The Dogmaticus*)
Elder Flowers

Fo-Ti-Tieng
Horseradish (Joseph Smith, *The Dogmaticus*)
Mustard Weed (Joseph Smith, *The Dogmaticus*)
Penny Royal
Peppermint
Poke Root (Joseph Smith, *The Dogmaticus*)
Prickly Ash (Joseph Smith, *The Dogmaticus*)
Rue
Spearmint
Yarrow

TONIC

Function – invigorating and strengthening to the body

Aspen
Balm Of Gilead (Joseph Smith, *The Dogmaticus*)
Barberry
Bayberry
Black Ader (Joseph Smith, *The Dogmaticus*)
Black Walnut
Boneset (small doses)
Bungle Weed
Burdock
Cascara Sagrada Bark
Chamomile
Chicory Root
Colombo (Joseph Smith, *The Dogmaticus*)
Dandelion Roots And Leaves
Eyebright

Fo-ti-tieng
Gentian (Joseph Smith, *The Dogmaticus*)
Hawthorne Berries
Kelp
Lady Slipper
Motherwort
Nettle

Periwinkle

Peruvian Bark (Benjamin Smith Barton, *Collection for an Easy Materia Medica,* Part I, 1798)

Poplar (Joseph Smith, *The Dogmaticus)*

Sassafras (Benjamin Smith Barton, *Collection for an Easy Materia Medica,* Part I, 1798)

Saw Palmetto

Skullcap

Unicorn Root (Joseph Smith, *The Dogmaticus)*

White Willow

Yarrow

Yellow Dock

VERMIFUGE

Function – expels worms

Aspen
Bearsfoot
Black Walnut
Blue Flag
Mandrake
Pink Root
Senna
Sorrel
Tansy
Wood Sage

Function – kills worms and parasites

Black Walnut
Kelp or Dulse
Pumpkin Seed
Wintergreen

HERBS

Agrimony

Digestive disorder
gastritis
jaundice
obstruction in liver
provokes urine
kills worms
strengthens lungs
William Cockburn (1669-1739) in *Account of Nature,* page 246, said that Agrimony is useful for dysentery.
Peter Smith, *Indian Doctor Dispense a Tory,* 1813:
    kidney
    bladder
    diabetes

Alfalfa

One of nature's finest herbs. Highly nutritive. Alkalize his body rapidly. Most effective Herb for arthritis.
Pituitary Hormone
Glands
High Food Values
Whooping Cough
Colds
Bladder
Kidneys
Bowels
Detoxifies Body
Liver
Promotes milk for nursing mothers

All Heal

Falling sickness
Kidney
Bladder
Colic
Kills Worms
Gout
Cramps

Epilepsy
Convulsions
Obstructions of Liver and Spleen
Itch
Stones
Toothache
Poison Bites
Expels Dead Birth (Culpeper)

Aloes

Expels pinworms
Cleans colon
Promotes menstruation
Cleans morbid matter from:
    Stomach
    Liver
    Kidneys
    Spleen
    Bladder
Sores on body
Hemorrhoids
Richard Blackmore (1650-1729) in *Discourse on Plague,* Part
    II, said that aloes is useful for plague.
B. Frank Scholl, *Library of Health,* 1925 edition:
    Laxative
    Colon
    Excites circulation of blood in pelvic area, promotes
        menstrual flow, used with iron and myrrh
    Avoid during pregnancy

In the Bible, **Proverbs 7:17** states:

*"I have perfumed my bed with myrrh, aloes, and
cinnamon."*

Song of Solomon 4:14 states:

"Spikenard and saffron; calamus and cinnamon, with all trees of frankincense; myrrh and aloes, with all the chief spices."

Angelica

Plague
All epidemics
Colic
Expels afterbirth
Stoppage of liver and spleen
Internal swelling
Gout
Toothache pain
Richard Blackmore (1650-1729) said in *Discourse on Plague,* Part II. that Angelica is useful for plague
William Salmon in *Family Dictionary* said that Angelica is useful in resisting plague.
Was in ancient times called Herb of the Holy Ghost or Herb of the Angels

Anise (Condiment)

Nausea
Colic
Gripping
Gas
B. Frank Scholl, *Library of Health,* 1925 edition:
Colic

Asparagus

William Salmon in *Family Dictionary,* page 28 said that Asparagus is useful for hip gout, gravel, kidney and bladder pain.

Aspen

Flu
Fever
Reduces pain of rheumatism
Colds
Headache pain
Neuralgia
Hay fever
Jaundice
Diabetes
Cancer
Sciatica pain
Cholera
Expels worms
Gas
Acid stomach
More valuable than aspirin without the side effects or upset
   stomach

Balsam Evergreen (Christmas tree)

Rheumatism
Kidney
Inflammation of bladder
Urinary problems

Barberry

Kidney
Nephritis
Jaundice
Gargle
Mouthwash
Cholera
Itch
Ringworm
B. Frank Scholl, *Library of Health,* 1924 edition:
   Kidneys

Blood disease
Gas
Liver
Constipation
Skin disease
Joseph Smith, *The Dogmaticus or Family Physician,* 1829:
  Digestion
  Improves appetite

Bay

Liver troubles
Pancreas
Spleen
Insect bites
Snake bite
Smallpox
Typhoid
Measles
Diphtheria
Nose or throat troubles
Berries:
  helpful when delivery is at hand
  Helps to expel afterbirth
  colds and fever

Bayberry

Sore throat
Gargle
Cleanse the stomach
Emetic
Goiter
Diarrhea or dysentery (when used in enema)
Gangrenous sores (poultice)
Boils, carbuncles
Infections (powder)
Jaundice
Canker sores

Flu
Fever
Cramps
Pain in stomach
Bronchitis
Used as tea for the old composition powder – as a tea or in milk
Digestive disorder
Hemorrhage
Joseph Smith, *The Dogmaticus or Family Physician,* 1829:
    Poultice for swellings
    Dysentery
Samuel Thomson, *New Guide to Health or Botanic Family physician,* 1833:
    Tooth Powder
    Scurvy
    Headache

Bearsfoot root

Liver
Spleen
Congestion of liver
Inflamed glands
Gas
Ointment

Beets

B. Frank Scholl, *Library of Health,* 1925 edition
    Gravel

Bethroot

Phelps Brown, *Complete Herbalist, People Their Own Physicians,* 1881:
    Bleeding from lungs
    Kidneys
    Coughs
    Asthma

    Ulcers
    Stings
    Bites

Betony

    Epilepsy
    Convulsions
    Coughs
    William Salmon in *Old Medical Instruments (1689)* Chapter 1, page 3, said that betony is useful for headaches.

Bitter Almonds

    William Salmon in *Old Medical Instruments (1689)*, Chapter 1, page 3, said that Bitter Almonds are useful for headaches.

Bitterroot

    Kidney
    Nephritis

Bittersweet

    Was used by ancients to remove witchcraft or spell
    Green berries are poison
    Use bark of root and twigs
    Leprosy
    Syphilis
    Ulcers
    Scrofula
    Eczema
    Glandular swelling
    Diarrhea
    Mucus in head
    Bladder
    Hemorrhage
    Hay fever
    Hemorrhoids

Fever
Meningitis
Typhoid
Whooping cough
Large doses causes vomiting and other side effects. Always use
in small dose. One of the best herbs to help swelling of glands.
Excellent as an ointment.

Black Cohosh

Cholera
Hysteria
St. Vitus dance
Epilepsy
Convulsions
Female – hormone
Uterine trouble
Relieves pain in childbirth – Taken when delivery is at hand
Relieves menstrual cramps
Rheumatism
Spinal meningitis
Asthma
Delirium tremens
Poison bites
High blood pressure
Coughs
Whooping cough
Liver and kidney problems
Dropsy
Phelps Brown, *Complete Herbalist, People Their Own
Physicians,* 1881:
Heart palpitations

Black Walnut

Leaves, bark and nut hulls
Green hulls contain organic iodine
Skin disease
Colitis

Expels tape worm
Diarrhea
Sore throat
Kills tuber bacillus
Kills malarial parasite
Lupus

Blue Cohosh

Regulates menstrual flow
Makes childbirth easy
Uterine problems
Rheumatism
Neuralgia
Inflammation of vagina
Cramps
Colic
Hysteria
Palpitations
High blood pressure
Whooping cough
Spasms
Epilepsy
Alkalize blood
Bronchial mucus

Blue Violet

Internal ulcers
Cancer
Skin disease
Skin cancer
Tumors
Gout
Coughs
Colds
Sore throat
Sores
Ulcers

Syphilis
Bronchitis
Nervousness
Gas
Causes perspiration

Boneset

Phelps Brown, *Complete Herbalist, People Their Own
    Physicians,* 1881:
    Typhoid
    Gas
    Flu

Borage

Inflamed eyes
Fever
Jaundice
Expels poisons
Snake, insect bites
Strengthens heart
Coughs
Itch
Ringworm
Sores
Ulcers
Nervousness

Buchu

Urinary organs
Relieves pain
Increases urine
Causes perspiration
Soothes enlargement of prostate
Soothes irritation of urethra
Kidney
Nephritis

B. Frank Scholl, *Library of Health,* 1925 edition
   Irritation of urinary organs
   Bladder
   Pain of urinating

Bungle weed

Coughs
Typhoid
Digestion
Increases appetite
Hemorrhage

Burdock

Purifies blood
Skin
Boils
Carbuncles
Increases flow of urine
Gout
Rheumatism
Burns
Wounds
Swelling
Hemorrhoids
Reduce weight
Swollen glands
Skin irritation
Wash for Burns
Relieves pain in bladder
Kidney stones
Acne
Eczema
Lupus
Psoriasis
Syphilis
Cancer
Leprosy

Tuberculosis
Powerful blood cleanser
Tonsil
Kidney and bladder
Gonorrhea
Canker sores
The ancients used it for skin disease. Has no equal for chronic skin problems.
B. Frank Scholl, *Library of Health,* 1925 edition
Venereal disease
Eliminating poison from blood
Phelps Brown, *Complete Herbalist, People Their Own Physicians,* 1881 said:
"This plant is too well known to be described."

Calamus Root

Fever
Stomach
Gas
Colic
Increases appetite
Destroys taste for tobacco
Bronchitis

Chamomile

General tonic
Increases appetite
Week stomach
Regulates menstruation
Kidney
Spleen
Colds
Bronchitis
Bladder troubles
Expels worms
Jaundice
Wash for weak or sore eyes

Sores
Wounds
Poultice for pain and swelling
Hysteria
Nervous disease
Gangrene
Typhoid
Aches
Pains
Colic
Increases urine
Promotes perspiration
Gas
Flu
Menstruation pain
William Salmon in *Old Medical Instruments* (1689), Chapter 1, Page 3, said that chamomile is useful for headaches.
Samuel Thomson, *New Guide to Health or Botanic Family physician,* 1833:
　　Removes calluses and corns

Cascara Sagrada

Laxative
Chronic constipation
Intestinal tonic
Gallstones
Increases bile
Liver
Digestive problems
Gas
Jaundice

Catnip

Convulsions
Relax
Spasms
Colic

Gas
Prevents gripping
Insanity
Fevers
Expels worms
Hysterical headache
Pain
Useful in enema
Epilepsy
Shock
Children and babies
Induces sleep
Acid stomach
Skin problems
Inflammation
Hysteria
Colds
Produces perspiration

Cayenne

Catalyst for all herbs
Yellow fever
Fever
Colds
Smoothes heart rhythm
Open wounds – stops bleeding
Stops internal bleeding
Rheumatism
Inflammation
Pleurisy
Kidney
Spleen
Pancreas
Lockjaw
Liniment
Pyorrhea
Old ulcers
Stimulant

Ulcerated stomach
Joseph Smith, *The Dogmaticus or Family Physician,* 1829
　　Stimulating, use as a bath for rheumatism with vinegar
Samuel Thomson, *New Guide to Health or Botanic Family physician,* 1833:
　　Used in all kinds of disease
　　Spotted fever
　　Glands
　　Saliva
　　Used with Lobelia

Cedron

Poison bites
Gas

Celandine

Skin
Eczema
Jaundice
Ringworm
Warts
Plague
Toothache
William Salmon in *Family Dictionary* said that Celandine is useful in resisting plague
William salmon in *Synopsis Medicinae* (1681), Page 629, said that Celandine is useful for eyes
Joseph Smith, *The Dogmaticus or Family Physician,* 1829:
　　Gravel
　　Dropsy
　　Spleen
Phelps Brown, *Complete Herbalist, People Their Own Physicians,* 1881:
　　Liver
　　Inflammation

Celery

Removes calcium deposits in joints
Arthritis
Gout
B. Frank Scholl, *Library of Health*, 1925 edition:
     Chronic rheumatism

Centaury

Epilepsy
Convulsions
Digestive disorder
Liver and gallbladder
Jaundice
Kills worms
Cramps
Gout
William Salmon in *Family Dictionary* said that Centaury leaves
     and flowers are useful in resisting plague.
William Salmon in *Family Dictionary* said that Centaury is
     useful for purging cholera, mucus, killing worms, healing
     wounds, and ulcers when applied to wounds. He stated that
     Galen has written a large treatise on Centaury (Page 69)

Cervi

William Beckett in *New Discoveries Relating to the Cure of
     Cancers* (1712), Page 30, said Cervi is useful for cancer.

Chamomile

Nervous stomach
Muscular pain
Strengthens body
Restores strength
Hysteria
poultice
Relieves pain
Joseph Smith, *The Dogmaticus or Family Physician*, 1829

Stomach
Indigestion
Loss of appetite
Fevers
Poultices for hardened tumors
Ointments for stiff joints

Chickweed

One of the best for external applications
Inflamed skin
Skin disease
Boils
Burns, scalds
Inflamed or sore eyes
Tumors
Piles
Cancer
Deafness
All kinds of wounds
Dissolves fat
Rheumatism
Stomach
Lungs
Poultice
Bowels
Bronchial inflammation
Erysipelas
Swollen testes
Ulcerated throat and mouth
Scurvy
Bronchitis
Red eyes (as a wash)
Ulcers
Sores
Peritonitis
Blood poisoning
Itching, burning genitals
Hemorrhoids

Chicory Root

Liver
Gout
Rheumatism

Chinchona Bark (Cleaves)

Kidney
Bladder
Burning urine
Fever
Scarlet fever
Measles
Acute disease
Skin diseases
Cancer
Eczema
Gonorrhea
Kidney stones
Scurvy
Water retention
Jaundice
Liver
Clean blood
Quinine used for malarial fever has a way of putting the parasites
    to sleep but does not stop the reoccurring fever. Quinine, like
    all other good Herb sources for synthetic drugs, finds itself
    classed among all dangerous drugs ending in "ine". Quinine
    can have some serious effects: ringing in the ears, dizziness,
    and it can even cause loss of hearing or death.

Citron

Richard Blackmore (1650-1729) in *Discourse on Plague,* Part II,
    that Syrup of Citron is useful for plague.

Cleavers

84

Bronchitis
Earache pain (drops in ears)
(Culpepper said this Herb was used to keep women lean and
 lank)
Phelps Brown, *Complete Herbalist, People Their Own
 Physicians,* 1881:
 Psoriasis
 Eczema
 Cancer
 Freckles
 Leprosy

Cleaves

Stones
Obstructions
Cleanse blood
Cancer

Clove

Toothache (oil of clove)
Richard Blackmore (1650-1729) in *Discourse on Plague,* Part II,
 said that Clove is useful for plague.

Coltsfoot

Joseph Smith, *The Dogmaticus or Family Physician,* 1829
 Coughs
 Consumption
 Dizziness
 Catarrh (mucus)

Colombo

Digestive disorder
Joseph Smith, *The Dogmaticus or Family Physician,* 1829:
 Gangrene

Cholera
Fever

Comfrey

Coughs
Catarrh
Inflammation of lung
Consumption
Hemorrhage
Asthma
Tuberculosis
Ulceration of kidneys
Ulceration of stomach or bowel
Blood in urine
Poultice
Bruises
Swelling
Sprains
Fractures
Relieves pain
Mucus in head
Anemia
Dysentery diarrhea
Inward bruises
Gangrenous sores
Wounds
Ulcers
Burns
Bronchial mucus
Bronchitis
Bone knitting qualities
Cancer
External use
Boils
Sores
William Salmon in *Family Dictionary* said that Comfrey is useful
for sprains.

William Cockburn (1669-1739) in *Account of Nature,* Page 246, said that Comfrey is useful for dysentery.

Phelps Brown, *Complete Herbalist, People Their Own Physicians,* 1881:
Bleeding lungs

Cranes Bill

William Cockburn (1669-1739) in *Account of Nature,* Page 246, said that Cranes Bill is useful for dysentery.

Daffodil

William Salmon, *Doron Medicum,* Chapter 1, verse 69, said Daffodil is useful for pain in joints.

Dandelion

Salad greens
Destroys acid in blood
Increases flow of urine
Jaundice
Skin disease
Scurvy
Eczema
Kidney
Diabetes
Dropsy
Fever
Inflammation of bowels
Female organs
Pancreas
Spleen
Gas
Rheumatism
Gout
Liver
Digestive disorder
Wash for sores

Ulcers

Obstructions of the liver, gallbladder, and spleen

One of the best herbs to clean the liver and gallbladder

High calcium food for people unable to take calcium in tablet

High in other minerals and vitamins

B. Frank Scholl, *Library of Health,* 1925 edition:

> Increases flow of urine
>
> Liver

Joseph Smith, *The Dogmaticus or Family Physician,* 1829:

> Opens urinary passages
>
> Removes obstructions

Echinacea

Blood poisoning

Peritonitis

Syphilis

Poison bites and stings

Swollen glands

Boils

Carbuncles

Fever

Gangrene

Tonsillitis

Pus formation

Sores

Infections

Wounds

Sore throat

Gargle

Eglantine

William Salmon in *Family Dictionary,* Page 257, said that Eglantine is useful for healing biting or mad dogs and for killing worms.

Elder

Twitching eyelids

Inflammation of eyes
Ointment: burns, scalds, skin disease
Tonic
Blood purifier
Cooling
Increases urine
Liver disease
Kidney disease
Erysipelas
Skin sores
Cold headache
Palsy
Rheumatism
Scrofula
Syphilis
Epilepsy
Dropsy
Semi-laxative
Flu
Cholera
One of the herbs well known and handed down through all ages
from Hippocrates
Flowers:
Bloodshot eyes
Sore eyes
Eyewash
Fever
Glandular swelling
Acid stomach
Acid skin
Cancer
Ulcers
Flu
Leaves – used as a poultice:
Skin
Itch
Acne
Wounds
Berries:

Fresh juice laxative
Cold
Sore throat
Chills
Promotes perspiration
Asthma
Bronchial mucus
Bark:
Water retention from heart or kidney
Epilepsy
Asthma
Liver
B. Frank Scholl, *library of health,* 1925 edition:
Flowers:
Rheumatism
Syphilis

Elecampane

Tuberculosis
Coughs
Asthma
Bronchitis
Lungs
Whooping cough
Retention of urine
Delayed menstruation
Kidney stones
Bladder
William Salmon in *Family Dictionary* said that Elecampane is useful for resisting plague

Evening Primrose

Liver
Gas
Asthma
Whooping cough

Eyebright

Eyes – inwardly and as a wash used with Goldenseal root

William salmon in *Synopsis Medicinae* (1681), Page 629, said that Eyebright is useful for eyes.

Phelps Brown, *Complete Herbalist, People Their Own Physicians,* 1881:

Coughs
Hoarseness
Earache
Headache

Fennel

Gas
Acid stomach
Gout
Colic
Cramps
Spasms
Snakebites
Insect bites
Food poison
Liver
Spleen
Jaundice
Increases urine
Increases menstrual flow
Eyewash
Gallbladder
Obesity (kills appetite)
Bronchitis

William Salmon in *Old Medical Instruments (1689)*, Chapter 1, Page 3, said that Fennell is useful for headaches.

William salmon in *Synopsis Medicinae* (1681), Page 69, said that Fennell is useful for eyes.

William Salmon in *Doctor Salmon's Last Legacy* stated in Chapter 1, that Fennell is used for eyes and states in Chapter 2

that in a tincture it takes away after birth and prevents
after pains
B. Frank Scholl, *Library of Health*, 1925 edition:
Colic
Cramps

Fenugreek

Poultice
Wounds
Inflammation
Fever
Lubricates intestines
William salmon in *Synopsis Medicinae* (1681), Page 69, said that
Fenugreek is useful for eyes.

Flaxseed

Poultices
Kidney inflammation
Ulcerated bowel
Ulcerated stomach
Bulk
B. Frank Scholl, *Library of Health*, 1925 edition:
Poultice
Boils
Abscesses
Inflammation of stomach
Burns (oil of flaxseed and linseed oil)

Fo-ti-tieng

Brain
Endocrine glands
Prevents senility
Rejuvenating influence on ductless glands
Promotes long life
Not a stimulant or irritant to sex centers but rather rejuvenator
and revitalizer of sexual glands

Fevers
Bowels
Skin
Brain

Gentian

Liver
Dysentery
Jaundice
Appetite
Increases circulation
Female organs
Fever
Colds
Gal
Convulsions
Gas
Expels worms
Menstrual cramps
Poison bites
William Salmon, *Doron Medicum,* (1644-1713), Chapter 1, Verse 14, said that Gentian is used for plague

Ginger

Root - chewed stimulates salivary glands
Paralysis of tongue
Sore throat
Diarrhea
Colds
Bronchitis
Gas
Cholera
Gout
Nausea
Menstrual cramps
Catalyst for all herbs to pelvic area
Bronchial mucus

William Salmon in *Old Medical Instruments (1689)*, Chapter 1, Page 3, said that Ginger is useful for headaches.

Ginseng

A preventative medicine
Promotes appetite
Digestive disturbances
Colds
Coughs
Constipation
Lung
Inflamed urinary tract
Produces perspiration if taken hot
Stomach troubles
Samuel Thomson, *New Guide to Health or Botanic Family physician,* 1833:
Nervine for nervous affections

Since the kingdom of vegetation for medicine has been cut off from past experience and in this generation left unexplored, we have lost much of the precious truth of the past.

The Chinese and Indian races have not lost their belief and knowledge of herbs as we have. The American Indian has maintained his knowledge of herbs also. It was known by all peoples of past history that herbs have the ability to repair deteriorated tissue, cleanse, and rejuvenate.

Ginseng has been used in old age for eyesight and nervous strain of years.

A man named Li Chung Yun, born in 1677, died in 1933 at the ripe old age of 256 years, according to official Chinese government records. He attributed his long life to a diet of fruit and herbs grown above the ground, with the exception of Ginseng. He also used other herbs and considered herbs to longevity like Fo-ti-tieng.

Ginseng has been used by the Chinese to allay fear assisting the nerve centers, increasing circulation to the brain, and overcoming nervous prostration. It was used as a general tonic, and they believed it developed character and fortitude as well as long life. They also believed that it reactivated the sex glands. When this Herb was used for over 5000 years in China by so many millions of people who had implicit faith in its restorative power, there has to be something Americans have not discovered about Ginseng. Leading medical doctors in China today still look upon Ginseng as a panacea and cure all, as well as a preventative medicine.

If it did not have some psychological effect, it would've been abandoned a long time ago. In the United States we plant and hunt for Ginseng and send thousands of dollars of this wonderful Herb to China almost with the attitude – because of the prejudice of American scientists – that if the superstitious Chinese want to buy this weed we will be glad to gather it for money – with an all-knowing smile of superiority. When all the time they are asking us to gather it, they do not tell us much about it, which makes me wonder just who is so smart. Then in turn we buy back their tannic acid tea and drink it with such stupid sophistication as should cause the Chinese to have the last laugh. The export and sale of Ginseng was once a capital crime in China and the use of the plant kept a guarded secret for thousands of years. When a soldier is wounded or fatigued from battle, the first thing he is given is Ginseng. A powerful antispasmodic, they give it for fatigue. It is useful in reflex nerve diseases, whooping cough, asthma, consumption, fevers, weaknesses of all kinds, and digestion.

The chief function of a Doctor in China was preventative rather than curative. Ginseng is still the most highly regarded and expensive botanical in the entire plant kingdom. It increases vigor of genital organs; vigor of gonads in a relationship to longevity.

The Greeks called Ginseng "plant of the sorcerers" and believed it possessed magical powers.

At night, as if it were singled out for us to notice, Ginseng gives off a phosphorescent glow. To approach a Ginseng plant at night causes the flowers to close and the glow is no longer visible. Plant hunters shoot arrows at the glow and find their arrows and the plant by daylight.

When we remove ourselves from the madness of drugs, we may find the therapeutic and rejuvenating properties of Ginseng and many others of nature's wonderful remedies.

Goldenrod

Cure-all type Herb

Goldenseal Root

Cure-all type Herb
Antibiotic: kills bacteria
Colds
Stomach and liver
Sores
Inflammation
Ringworm
Erysipelas
Skin disease
Nausea in pregnancy
Ulcerated stomach bowel
Pyorrhea
Diabetes: acts like insulin
Diabetic sores
Wounds
Burns
Bleeding bladder
Internal bleeding
Duodenal ulcers
Sore eyes
Chronic mucus
Enlarged spleen
Nose, throat
Bronchial tubes
Intestinal trouble
Heals mucous membrane anywhere in the body

Bronchitis
Hemorrhage
Typhoid fever
Samuel Thomson, *New Guide to Health or Botanic Family physician,* 1833:
Weak stomach
Restores digestive power

Gotu-Kola

Mental troubles
Blood pressure
Abscesses
Bruises
Swollen parts
Rheumatic swelling
Fever
Powder healing on ulcers
Memory improvement
Energy
Overcomes brain fatigue
Rheumatism
Neuritis
Nervous breakdown
Invaluable brain food for learned professionals
Clear voice
Promotes longevity
Prevents senility
Endocrine glands
Strengthens heart

Gravel Root

Kidney stones

Hawthorne Berries

Heart
Unstoppable for heart disease

Use with Vitamin E

Herbane

William Salmon, *Doron Medicum,* (1644-1713) Chapter 1, Verse 47, said that Herbane is useful for diabetes.

Hops

Nervine
Induces sleep
Delirium tremens
Toothache
Earache
Neuralgia
Increases urine
Tones liver
Helps excessive sex desire
Gonorrhea
Inflammation
Boils
Tremors
Swelling
Old ulcers
Epilepsy
Convulsions
Shock
B. Frank Scholl, *Library of Health,* 1925 edition:
Poultice local pain
Gonorrhea
Delirium tremens
Settles stomach
Insomnia
Restlessness
Phelps Brown, *Complete Herbalist, People Their Own Physicians,* 1881:
Anxiety
Exhaustion
Horehound

Bronchitis
Produces perspiration if taken hot
Laxative
Gas
Jaundice
Asthma
Hysteria
Expels worms
Sore throat
Coughs
Consumption
Croup

Horse-Radish

Joseph Smith, *The Dogmaticus or Family Physician,* 1829
Palsy
Dropsy
Scurvy
Rheumatism
Fever
Steeped in vinegar removes freckles and ring worms

Horsetail

Cure-all type herbs
Kidney
Bladder
Gas
Helps to utilize calcium
Mucus
Pus
Glands
Skin
Ulcers
Hemorrhage
Stops bleeding external or internal
Nosebleed

Where worms were parasites have been killed, Horsetail herb
will expel them from the body.

Hyacinth

Richard Blackmore (1650-1729) in *Discourse on Plague,* Part II,
said that Hyacinth is useful for plague.

Hyssop

Bronchitis
Bruises
Colds
Asthma
Lung
Fever
Kidney and bladder
Reduces blood pressure
Jaundice
Fluid buildup
Coughs
Expels worms
Kills body lice
Eye trouble
Joseph Smith, *The Dogmaticus or Family Physician,* 1829:
    Whooping cough
    Consumption
In the Bible, Exodus 12:22 says that Hyssop or Marjoram is
dipped in blood and placed on door.
In the Bible, Psalm 51:7 talks about purging with hyssop.

Juniper

Formula:
    Peach leaves
    Marshmallow
    Juniper
Stomach
Colic

Expels gas

Coughs

Short breath

Cramps

Convulsions

Brain

Oil or wash for insect bites

Snake and dog bites

Consumption

Delivery

Strengthening to nerves

Gout

Sciatica

Rheumatism

Pain

Diabetes

Gargle

Strengthens gums

Kills worms

Leper sores

Itch

Palsy

Plague

Kidney

Nephritis

William Salmon in *Family Dictionary* (1644), page 257, said that Juniper berries are useful for increased flow of urine, for gravel, stones, colds, disease of brain, future fixation, to help digestion, kills worms, expel wind, and formalities of the bowel.

B. Frank Scholl, *Library of Health,* 1925 edition:

Bright's disease

Joseph Smith, *The Dogmaticus:*

Oil clears the urinary passage

Lady Slipper

Neuralgia pain

Promotes sleep

Hysteria
Relieves nervous headaches
Epilepsy
Convulsions
Shock

Laudanum

In the Bible, Laudanum is called a balm.

Today we call it opium.

A tincture of opium was first prepared by Paracelsus. Pure opium powder is seldom used in drug medicine.

Morphine is made from the most important alkaloid found in opium.

Heroin is a drug made from morphine but much more poisonous and habit-forming. All the drugs used today which end in "ine" are the dangerous alkaloids whose source began originally with organic plants. Some are made synthetically so as to be produced more cheaply with greater allowable profits.

These alkaloids have been used among physicians since time began. There is great danger in overdose. These dangerous herbs have both blessed and cursed mankind in all generations of time.

It is my opinion that the plant alkaloid causes such a rapid change to an alkaline condition that it causes insensibility and in high doses can kill. If we could learn to live in a cleaner, physical state we would suffer less pain and have no need of the opiates or the synthetic drugs created by man.

Lemon

William Salmon stated in *Practice of Physick* (1707) that Lemon is helpful for rheumatism.

William Salmon states in *Practice of Physick*, 2nd Edition (1707), Page 49, that the juice of Lemon is useful for scarlet fever.

B. Frank Scholl, *Library of Health*, 1925 edition:
Anti-narcotic
Asthma

Antidote in alkaline poisoning
Biliousness
Corns
Coughs
Colds
Hoarseness
Sore throat
Dropsy
Erysipelas
Fevers
Headache
Rheumatism
Gout
Scarlet fever
Malarial disease
Hemorrhages
Itching of anus
Jaundice
La Grippe
Scurvy
Syphilis
Remove tan from face
Vomiting

Licorice

Bronchitis
Acts as natural cortisone or cortin hormone
Hypoglycemia
Hyperglycemia
Adrenal exhaustion
Addison's disease
Cushing's disease
(Refer to my book *Is Any Sick Among You?*)
William Salmon in *Family Dictionary* said that Licorice is
    useful in resisting plague.

Lilies
Throat

Mouth

Sore eyes

Lockjaw

Sores

Gonorrhea

William salmon stated in *Practice of* (1707) that Lilies are helpful for rheumatism.

William salmon, *Doron Medicum,* (1644-1713), Chapter 1, Verse 56, said that Lily is useful to cure burning.

William Cockburn (1669-1739) in *Account of Nature,* Page 246, aid that Water Lilies are useful for dysentery.

B. Frank Scholl, *Library Of Health,* 1925 edition: Heart (small doses – strengthens; large doses – quiets) Palpitations

Lobelia

Most powerful relaxant

Emetic when taken

Best used with other herbs

Excellent for poultices

Reduces heart palpitations

Fevers

Pneumonia

Meningitis

Pleurisy

Peritonitis

Removes obstructions in body

Lung

Whooping cough

Rheumatism

Canker

Spasms

Lockjaw

Convulsions

Seizures

Antispasmodic

Weak heart

Laryngitis

Angina pectoris

In large doses it relaxes and should then be followed by a
stimulant such as Cayenne.
Strengthens muscle action
Difficulty breathing
Asthma
Chickenpox
Measles
Smallpox
Scarlet fever
One of the most valuable botanicals
Epilepsy
Bronchial mucus
Shock
Ointment
Benjamin Smith Barton, *Collection for an Easy Materia Medica,*
Part I, 1798:
Syphilis
Gonorrhea
Samuel Thomson, *New Guide to Health or Botanic Family
physician,* 1833:
Nervousness
Small doses: it acts like a relaxant
Large doses: it acts like an emetic
Should always be used with cayenne
Hydrophobia

Madenhair

William Salmon, *Doron Medicum,* (1644-1713) Chapter 1, Verse
4, stated that Madenhair is useful for opening obstructions,
lungs, and provoking urine.

Mallow

Lung
throat
mucus
diarrhea
douche

sore eyes (bathe)

pneumonia

kidney disease

William Salmon, *Doron Medicum,* (1644-1713), Chapter 1, 1st 8, said that Mallow is useful for pain of stone, bladder.

William Salmon in *Old Medical Instruments (1689)*, Chapter 1, Page 3, said Mallow is useful for headaches.

William Salmon in *Synopsis Medicinae* (1681), Page 629, said Mallow is useful for eyes.

Mandrake

Stimulates glands to help the action

Powerful intestinal cleanser – laxative

Overcomes adhesions

Overcomes anti-intoxication

Overcomes putrefaction and decaying fecal wastes adhering to intestinal wall

Liver

Rheumatism

Biliousness

Mandrake has been called "Herb of the sorcerers"

Uterine diseases

Jaundice

Fever

Useful with Herb formulas

Joseph Smith, *The Dogmaticus or Family Physician,* 1829:
  Asthma
  Coughs
  Consumption
  Venereal disease
  Destroys worms

In the Bible, Genesis 30:14 states:
  "And Reuben went in the days of wheat harvest, and found mandrakes in the field, and brought them unto his mother Leah. Then Rachel said to Leah, Give me, I pray the, of thy son's mandrakes."

In the Bible, Of Solomon 7:13 States:

"The mandrakes give a smell, and at our gates are all manner of pleasant fruits, new and old, which I have laid up for the, o my beloved."

Phelps Brown, *Complete Herbalist, People Their Own Physicians,* (1881) said:
"In constipation, it acts upon the bowels without disposing them to subsequent costiveness."

Marigold

Richard Blackmore (1650-1729) in *Discourse on Plague,* Part II, that Marigold flowers are useful for plague.

William Salmon in *Family Dictionary* said that Marigold is useful for resisting plague.

Marjoram

Sour stomach
Loss of appetite
Cough
Consumption
Spleen
Suppressed menstruation
Poison bites
Edema
Scurvy
Itch
Jaundice
Deafness
Toothache
Headache
Indigestion

A condiment Herb – you can see why it would be helpful added to food as a flavoring.

In the Bible, Exodus 12:22 it says that Hyssop or Marjoram, dip in blood and placed on door.

William Salmon, *Doron Medicum,* (1644-1713) stated in Chapter 1, that Sweet Marjoram could be used after surgery on a tumor as a poultice of leaves and roots.

Marshmallow

Inflammation
Lung
Mucus
Diarrhea
Dysentery
Douche
Irritation of vagina
Pneumonia
Kidney disease
Nephritis
Gastritis
Kidney stones
Bronchitis
B. Frank Scholl, *Library of Health,* 1925 edition:
   Dressing for skin disease
   Bright's disease
   Lung
   Inflammation of kidney and bladder

Meadowsweet

Kidney stones

Melilat

William Salmon in *Synopsis Medicinae* (1681), Page 69, said that
   Melilat is useful for eyes.

Mexican Damiana

Sexual glands
Overcomes impotence
Brain
Nerves
Gonads
Overcomes loss of nerve

Energy to limbs
Bladder ailments
Nephritis

Mistletoe

Cholera
Nervine
Epilepsy
Convulsions
Hysteria
Delirium
Nervousness
Heart trouble
Shock

Motherwort

Longevity herb
Heart
The best Herb in the herbal kingdom to promote menstruation
Strengthens female genital organs
Strengthens the womb
Useful during pregnancy
Muscle spasms
Twitching muscles
Calms heart and nerves
William Salmon, *Doron Medicum* (1644-1713), Chapter 1, Verse
21, said that Motherwort is useful for convulsions, sores and
healing skin.

Mugwort

Female problems
Gravel
Kidney stones
Increases urine flow
Fever
Gout

Bruises
Abscesses
Carbuncles
Rheumatism
Pain in stomach
Pain in bowels
William Salmon in *Family Dictionary* said that Mug wort is good for yellow jaundice and in resisting plague.
William Salmon in *Old Medical Instruments (1689)*, Chapter 1, page 3, said that Mugwort is useful for headaches.

Mullein

Asthma (fumes)
Croup
Bronchitis
Bleeding of lung
Difficulty breathing
Hay fever
Throat gargle
Washing of open sores
Inflammation
Swollen testicles or scrotum
Ulcers
Tonsils
Mumps
Glandular swelling
Sore throat
Swollen joints
Mucus
Bleeding bowels
Hemorrhage
Coughs
Colds
Diarrhea
External skin irritation
Oil of mullein for inflammation of inner ear
Earache
Used internally or externally

Tuberculosis
Pleurisy
Burns
Wounds
Bone diseases
Skin diseases
B. Frank Scholl, *Library of Health*, 1925 edition:
  Lungs
  Diarrhea
  Inflammation of bladder

Mustard

Emetic: produces vomiting
Not good as a food
Poultice:
  If egg white is used with flour instead of water it will not
  blister
Foot bath

Myrrh

Mouthwash
Excellent in ointments
Bronchial and lung disease
Pyorrhea
Sore mouth
Sore throat
Best added in small amounts to formulas
Washing sores or powder
Antibiotic on open wounds
Diphtheria
Ulcerated throat
Bronchitis
Typhoid fever
Richard Blackmore (1650-1729) in *Discourse on Plague,* Part ii,
  said that Myrrh is useful for plague.
In the Bible, Song of Solomon 1:13, Myrrh is used as part of love
  expression.

In the Bible, Genesis 37:25 states:
> "And they sat down to eat bread: and they lifted up their eyes and looked, and, behold, a company of Ishmaelites came from Gilead with their camels bearing spicery and balm and myrrh, going to carry it down to Egypt."

In the Bible, Genesis 43:11 states:
> "And their father Israel said unto them, If *it must be* so now, do this; take of the best fruits in the land in your vessels, and carry down the man a present, a little balm, and a little honey, spices, and myrrh, nuts, and almonds"

Phelps Brown, *Complete Herbalist, People Their Own Physicians,* 1881:

Asthma

Gangrenous ulcers

Gums

Teeth

Samuel Thomson, *New Guide to Health or Botanic Family physician,* 1833:

Wounds

Old sores

Nettle

Kidney trouble

Expels gravel

Increases flow of urine

Green poultice – relieves pain (left too long will raise blister)

Increases menstrual flow

Kills worms

Obesity combined with other herbs

Fever

Colds

Applied externally stops bleeding

Mucus

Lungs

Stomach

Blood purifier

Neuralgia

Coughs

Shortness of breath
Has the ability to expel mucus
Inflammation
Arthritis, rheumatoid
Lupus
Anemia
Asthma
Hemorrhage of lungs
Tuberculosis
Headache
Whooping cough
Sore throat
Gout
Burns
Bee sting
William Salmon in *Family Dictionary*, Page 339, said that Nettle juice is useful for stopping bleeding, pain in head, being drunk, provokes urine, and for application to tumors and inflammation.
B. Frank Scholl, *Library of Health,* 1925 edition:
Hemorrhage
Nosebleed
Lungs
Intestines
Urinary organs

Oak Leaves

William Cockburn (1669-1739) in *Account of Nature,* Page 246, said that Oak Leaves are useful for dysentery.

Olive Oil

B. Frank Scholl, *Library of Health,* 1925 edition:
constipation
gallstones
digestion
scalp treatment

used by swimmers to rub on body, to endure greater cold and withstand fatigue

Onion

B. Frank Scholl, *Library of Health,* 1925 edition:
Poultice for burns or scalds
Bronchitis
Croup
Constipation
Joseph smith, *The Dogmaticus or Family Physician,* 1829:
Internal abscesses

Opiates

William Salmon stated in *Practice of Physick* (1707), 2nd Edition, Page 49, that Opiates are useful for scarlet fever.

Parsley

Increases flow of urine
Jaundice
Fever
Stones – kidney
Gallstones
Liver
Spleen
Preventative medicine
Cancer
Syphilis
Gonorrhea
High potassium
Insect bites
Stings
Fomentations
Poultice for swollen glands
Kidney
Bladder

William Salmon in *Family Dictionary*, Page 366, said that Parsley diminishes milk of women.

B. Frank Scholl, *Library of Health*, 1925 edition:
Scant menstruation
Relieves pain

Peach

Laxative
Nervous system
Whooping cough
Stomach troubles
Jaundice
Expels worms
Cholera
Bladder
Uterine troubles
Morning sickness – pregnancy
Fever
Powdered leaves heals sores and wounds
Worms
Gas
Bronchitis

William Salmon in *Family Dictionary*, Page 370, said that Peach Flowers Syrup is useful for colick or belly ache, gripping, that it purges well and pleasantly, and that it kills worms.

William Salmon in *Old Medical Instruments* (1689), Chapter 1, page 3, said that Peach kernels are useful for headaches.

B. Frank Scholl, *Library of Health*, 1925 edition:
Leaves:
Jaundice
Worms

Pennyroyal

Epilepsy
Convulsions
Fever
Gout

Jaundice

Promotes perspiration

William Salmon in *Family Dictionary*, Page 373 said that Pennyroyal is useful for coughs, colds, jaundice, dropsy, stones or gravel, and hoarseness.

B. Frank Scholl, *Library of Health*, 1925 edition:

Gas

Colic

Obnoxious to mosquitoes

Peony

Epilepsy

William Salmon in *Family Dictionary* said that Peony is useful for resisting plague.

B. Frank Scholl, *Library of Health*, 1925 edition:

Spasm

Whooping cough

Nervous disease

Epilepsy

Most of the old books mentioned Peony for brain problems. It is an herb we should learn more about.

Phelps Brown, *Complete Herbalist, People Their Own Physicians,* (1881) agreed with the above.

Peppermint

Chills

Dizziness

Gas

Nausea

Vomiting

Diarrhea

Dysentery

Cholera

Heart trouble

Palpitations

Influenza

Hysteria
Rheumatism
Neuralgia
Headache
Insanity
Convulsions and spasms in babies
Sudden fainting
Coldness
Pale
One of the best stimulants
Brings back normal body warmth
Gripping pain
Strengthens heart
Cleanses and strengthens entire body
Better than aspirin for headache
Strengthens nerves
Assists digestion
Colic
Shock
One of the best stimulants
Oil and menthol used externally for:
  Rheumatism
  Neuralgia
  Toothache
Internally:
  Fainting
  Dizzy
  Extreme coldness
  Pale countenance
B. Frank Scholl, *Library of Health,* 1925 edition:
  Seasickness
  Nausea
  Vomiting
  Colic

Periwinkle

Diabetes

William Cockburn (1669-1739) in *Account of Nature,* page 246, said that Periwinkle is useful for dysentery.

B. Frank Scholl, *Library of Health,* 1925 edition:
Mucus
Diarrhea
Hemorrhage
Gargle and mouthwash for spongy gums

Peruvian Bark

Benjamin Smith Barton, *Collection for an Easy Materia Medica,* Part I, 1798:
Fever

Pink Root

Roundworms
(not to be used alone)
B. Frank Scholl, *Library of Health,* 1925 edition:
Worms
Used with Senna

Plantain

Bleeding
Wounds
Swollen glands
Pain in bowels
Mucus in head
Kills worms
Sore eyes
Water retention
External wash for:
Itch
Ring worms
Running sores
Burns
Scales
Ulcers

Eczema
Colitis
Nausea
Gas

William Cockburn (1669-1739) in *Account of Nature,* page 246, said that Plantain so for dysentery.

B. Frank Scholl, *Library of Health,* 1925 edition:
  Applied to skin checks bleeding

Pleurisy Root

Bronchial mucus
Typhoid fever
Promotes perspiration
Pleurisy
Colds
Bronchial problems
Scarlet fever
Rheumatic fever
Lung
Measles
Suppressed menstruation
Dysentery
Kidneys
Asthma

Poke Root

Tonic
Enlarged glands
Spleen, thyroid
Hard deliver
Biliousness
Inflammation
Kidney
Lymphatic glands
Goiter
Poultice and liniment
Skin disease

Syphilis
Eczema
Itch
Poultice for caked breasts
Especially helpful in formula
Ulcers
Ringworm
Rheumatism
Gas

Poplar (Quaking Aspen)

Rheumatism
Fever
Pain
Neuralgia
Kidney
Diabetes
Hay fever
Will expel worms
External wash for:
  Cancer
  Ulcers
  Gangrenous wounds
  Eczema
  Burns
  Gonorrhea
  Syphilis
  Jaundice

Potato

B. Frank Scholl, *Library of Health,* 1925 edition:
Swelling
Muscles
Joints
Lumbago
Relieves pain externally

Prickly Ash Bark

Chewing helps
Sores in mouth and tooth
Aches
Used for all diseases
Female
Increases saliva
Paralysis of tongue
Cholera
Blood purifier
Wounds and skin ulcers
Joseph Smith, *The Dogmaticus or Family Physician,* 1829:
    Toothache
    Rheumatism
    Venereal ulcers
Samuel Thomson, *New Guide to Health or Botanic Family physician,* 1833:
    Fever
    Sleepiness and lethargy

Pulsatilla

Menstrual difficulties from exhaustion

Pumpkin Seeds

Excellent used in formula to remove parasites
Salmonella
Trichinosis
Roundworms
Pinworms
B. Frank Scholl, *Library of Health,* 1925 edition:
    Removal of tapeworm used with castor oil and turpentine

Psyllium

Colitis
Ulcers

Hemorrhoids
Anti-intoxication
Adheres to and removes putrefaction and hardened waste from
colon
Intestinal Tract:
    Healing
    Bulk agent
    Lubricates
    Moistens
    Heals

Queen of the Meadow

Kidney
Nephritis
Diarrhea
Edema
Neuralgia
Rheumatism
Sores
Joseph Smith, *The Dogmaticus or Family Physician,* 1829:
    Gravel
    Dropsical disease

Quercetain

William Beckett in *New Discoveries Relating to the Cure of
Cancers* (1712), page 30, said Quercetain is useful for cancer.

Red Clover

Cancer
Leprosy
Blood purifier
Wounds
Nerves
Bronchial
Whooping cough
Syphilis

Douche
Skin cancer
Skin disease
Blood disease
Leukemia (cancer)

Red Raspberry

Cankers
Diarrhea – infants
Decrease menstrual flow
Will allay nausea
Pregnancy
Anti-acid
Digestive disorders
Gastritis
Fever
Best known agent for child bearing
Prevents miscarriage
Easy parturition at birth
Enrich milk
Nausea in pregnancy
Prolapses of uterus
Sustaining to nerves
High mineral and vitamin source

Rosemary

Colds
Colic
Nervousness
Headache
Mouthwash – foul breath
Sore throat
Coughs
Consumption
Strengthens eyes
William Salmon stated in *Practice of Physick* (1707) that
    Rosemary is helpful for rheumatism.

William Salmon in *Family Dictionary* said that Rosemary is useful to resist plague.

B. Frank Scholl, *Library of Health,* 1925 edition:
Ointment for neuralgia
Chronic rheumatism
Lumbago

Rue

(Do not boil)
Congestion of uterus
Suppressed menstruation
Stomach
Bowel cramps
Nervousness
Worms
Confused mind
Insanity
Colic
Convulsions
Pain in head
Dizziness
Counter poison
Snake – insect bites
Hysteria
Swollen testicles
Poison bites

Saffron

Breaks out measles, skin diseases, etc.
Scarlet fever
Produces profuse perspiration when taken hot
Regulates menstrual flow
Hysteria
Neutralizes uric acid
Gout
Acid stomach
Fever
Hypoglycemia

Hyperglycemia

Cushing's disease

William Salmon in *Family Dictionary* said that Saffron is good for yellow jaundice.

William Salmon in *Family Dictionary* also said that it is restorative but taking too much of it is troublesome to the spirit.

In this same book, Salmon also stated that Saffron is helpful for weak stomach, faintness of heart; that taken with wine it prevents drunkenness, and that it heals bites of serpent and spider.

Henry Burdon (1743) in *The Fountain of Health*, page 13, said that Saffron, Peony, Water, Black cherry are useful to correct acidity in stomach.

William Salmon stated in *Practice of Physick* (1707) that Saffron is helpful for rheumatism.

William Salmon stated in *Practice of Physick* (1707) page 49, that Saffron is useful for scarlet fever.

William Cockburn (1669-1739) in *Account of Nature,* page 246, said that Saffron is useful for dysentery.

B. Frank Scholl, *Library of Health,* 1925 edition:

Causes sweating

Rheumatism

Measles

Scarlet fever

In the Bible, Of Solomon 4:14 States:

spikenard and saffron; calamus and cinnamon, with all trees of frankincense; myrrh and aloes, with all the chief spices.

Sage

Digestion

Ulcerated throat or mouth

Excessive sexual desire

Gas

Expels worms

Stops bleeding (wounds)

Liver

Kidney

Nervousness
Fever
Removes dandruff
Substitute for quinine
Pneumonia
Hair rinse
Improves circulation
Stops milk flow for weaning
William Salmon, *Doron Medicum,* (1644-1713), chapter 1, verse 92, states that Sage prevents miscarriages.
William Salmon in *Family Dictionary*, page 442, said that Sage is useful for colds, mucus, falling sickness, and pains in joints. In the same book he said that it is useful to resist plague.

St. John's Wort

Phelps Brown, *Complete Herbalist, People Their Own Physicians,* 1881:
Hemorrhage
Palsy
Sciatica

Salep

Used in ancient love potions
Sexual glands
Endocrine glands
Used to restore youth

Sanicle

Powerful Herb classed as a cure-all
Internally and externally
Mucus
Gargle
Colds
Sore throat
Cleanses system
Ulcers

Stomach

Lungs, consumption

Gonorrhea

Syphilis

Kidneys

Throat irritations

William Cockburn (1669-1739) in *Account of Nature,* page 246, said that Sanicle is useful for dysentery.

Culpepper says it heals wounds, chapter hands.

An old Italian proverb said:
"He that has Self-heal and Sanicle needs no other physician."

Benjamin Smith Barton, *Collection for an Easy Materia Medica,* Part I, (1798):
Cancer

Sarsaparilla

Male hormone

Rheumatism

Gout

Skin eruptions

Ringworm

Antidote for poison

Mucus

Fever

Colds

Gas

Infants infected with venereal

Sarsaparilla Root (Honduras)

Rejuvenating spring tonic

Blood purifier

Rheumatic affections

Venereal disease

Skin disease

Contains substances known as saponins which are another source of male sex hormone – testosterone

Rejuvenating effect on gonads

Sassafras

Purifies blood
Cleanse system
Stomach
Bowel
Relieves gas
Spasms
Wash for inflamed eyes
Kidneys
Bladder
Chest
Throat troubles
Oil of Sassafras:
    Toothache
    Varicose ulcers
William Beckett in *New Discoveries Relating to the Cure of Cancers* (1712), page 30, said Sassafras is useful for cancer.
Benjamin Smith Barton, *Collection for an Easy Materia Medica,* Part I, (1798):
    Fever

Saw Palmetto

Wasting disease
Glandular tissue
Increasing flesh rapidly
Builds strength
Stimulates assimilation
Tonic to nerves and all mucous membrane
Overcomes nasal congestion and congestion of ear passages
Atrophy of testes, mammary glands

Skullcap

Nerve tonic – one of the best herbs for the nervous system
Delirium tremens
Produces sleep

Palsy
Convulsions
Epilepsy
Rheumatism
Poison bites
Suppress undue sex desire
Hysteria
Rickets
Cholera
Shock
B. Frank Scholl, *Library of Health,* 1925 edition:
   Delirium tremens
   Nervous exhaustion
   Epilepsy

Self-Heal

Italian proverb:
   "He that has Self-heal and Sanicle needs no other physician."
Convulsions
Liver
Expels worms
Stops bleeding
Ulcers in mouth
Genital ulcers
Cure-all type of Herb

Senna

Laxative
Worms
Halitosis
Biliousness
William Salmon in *Old Medical Instruments (1689)*, Chapter 1, page 3, said that Senna is useful for headaches.

Shavegrass

Gout

Slippery Elm

Bowel – colitis
Bladder problems
Lung troubles
Diarrhea
Ulcerated stomach
Boils
Inflammation
Bronchitis
Female problem – as suppository
Excellent poultice
Gastritis

Snakeroot

William Salmon stated in *Practice of Physick* (1707) 2nd edition, page 49, that Snakeroot is useful for scarlet fever.

Snakeweed

Richard Blackmore (1650-1729) in *Discourse on Plague,* Part II, that Snakeweed is useful for plague.

Solomon's Seal

External
Bruises
Female
Poison ivy
Pain

Spearmint

Colic
Gas
Bowels
Spasms

Water retention
Nausea
Vomiting
Gravel in bladder
Suppressed, painful urine
Digestion
Settle stomach
Obstructions of liver
Thins blood
Shock
Soothes nerves
Stops vomiting in pregnancy

Spikenard

Easy childbirth
Shortens labor
Blood purifier
Venereal disease
Coughs
Colds
Chest infections
William Salmon, *Doron Medicum,* (1644-1713), Chapter 1, verse 70, states that Spikenard is useful for women with child. Use with cinnamon, nutmeg, and cloves to cure palpitations, jaundices, and apoplexy. It comforts brain and nerves.
In the Bible, Song of Solomon 1:2 states that Spikenard is used as perfume.

Squaw Vine (Brigham Tonic)

Makes childbirth easy
Sore eyes (wash)
Urinary troubles
Increases menstrual flow
Sore nipples (wash)
Kills germs
Syphilis
Asthma

Bronchial
Lungs
Headaches
Fever
Skin
Kidney and bladder
Arthritic pain
Rheumatic pain
Gonorrhea
Delayed menstruation

Stillengia

Like Lobelia in large doses causes vomiting and purging.

Tansy

Kidney
Nephritis
Colds
Fever
Gas
Expels worms
Hysteria
Jaundice
Edema
Kidney
Weak veins
Palpitations of heart
Samuel Thomson, *New Guide to Health or Botanic Family physician,* 1833:
  For stoppage of urine

Thyme

Colic
Gas
cough
Whooping cough

Spasms
Bronchial irritation
Promotes perspiration

Tormentils Root

Richard Blackmore (1650-1729) in *Discourse on Plague,* Part II,
said that Tormentils Root is useful for plague.

William Cockburn (1669-1739) in *Account of Nature,* page 246,
said that roots of Tormentil are useful for dysentery.

Uva Ursi

Kidneys
Nephritis
Diabetes
Dysentery
Spleen
Liver
Bladder
Gonorrhea

Valerian

Nerve tonic
Measles
Scarlet fever
Colic
Convulsions
Fever
Colds
Gas
Sores
Pimples
Hysteria
Pain
Promotes sleep
Not a narcotic
Shock
Epilepsy

B. Frank Scholl, *Library of Health,* 1925 edition:
Nervous disorder
Nervous headache
Hysteria
Convulsions
Whooping cough
Joseph Smith, *The Dogmaticus or Family Physician,* 1829
Fits
Spasms

Vervain

Produces profuse perspiration
Fever
Colds
Whooping cough
Pneumonia
Consumption
Asthma
Expels mucus from throat and chest
Increases menstrual flow
Skin disease
Expels worms
Insanity
Nervousness
Headache
Lung infections
Liver, spleen
Coughs
Epilepsy
Wheezing
William Salmon in *Old Medical Instruments (1689)*, Chapter 1,
    page 3, said that Vervain is useful for headaches.

Vinegar

Richard Blackmore (1650-1729) in *Discourse on Plague,* Part II,
    said that Vinegar is useful for plague.

Violet

Headache
Cancer

Ulcers
Bedsores
Produces perspiration
Whooping cough
Bronchitis
Coughs
Inflammation
 of eyes
Heart
Nerves
William Salmon, *Doron Medicum,* (1644-1713), Chapter III, verse 7, that Violet is helpful for headache.
William Salmon stated in *Practice of Physick* (1707) that Violet is helpful for rheumatism.

White Ash

Joseph Smith, *The Dogmaticus or Family Physician,* 1829:
Promotes perspiration
Resists poison
Cathartic

White Willow

Dim eyesight
Cataracts
Stomach troubles
Sour stomach
Heartburn
Fever
Chills
Rheumatism
Gangrene
Cancer

Eczema
Stops bleeding
Anti-emetic
Eyewash

Wild Carrot

Kidney
Nephritis
Kidney stones
Antibiotic
Flu
Colds

Wild Lettuce

William Salmon, *Doron Medicum,* (1644-1713) said in Chapter
1, verse 50, that Wild Lettuce is helpful for gonorrhea and for
causing sleep.

Wild Yam

Cholera
Neuralgia
Pregnancy pain
Allay nausea
Cramps during pregnancy
Helps to prevent miscarriages
Liver
Spasms
Rheumatic pains
Nerves
Expels gas
Urinary tract
Cortisone is made from the Wild Yam
Natural Cortin hormone
Hypoglycemia
Hyperglycemia
Cushing's disease

Addison's disease
B. Frank Scholl, *Library of Health,* 1925 edition:
   Appendicitis

Wintergreen

Gonorrhea
Obstruction in bowel
Diabetes
Catarrh of bladder
Sciatica
Skin diseases
Inflammatory rheumatism
Rheumatic fever
Stimulates heart, stomach and respiration
Kills parasites
Large doses causes vomiting
Small doses kill parasites
Aids digestion
William Cockburn (1669-1739) in *Account of Nature,* page 246,
   said that Wintergreen is useful for dysentery.
B. Frank Scholl, *Library of Health,* 1925 edition:
   Rheumatism

Wood Betony

Applied externally
Wounds heal and close rapidly
Old ulcers
Bring forth splinters
Headache
Insanity
Neuralgia
Heartburn
Indigestion
Stomach cramps
Jaundice
Parkinson's disease
Convulsions

Gout
Colic
Edema
Colds
Worms
Poison bites
Phelps Brown, *Complete Herbalist, People Their Own Physicians,* 1881:
Earache
Kidney obstructions
Coughs
Gas
Stops bleeding
Mouth and nose

Wood Sorrel

Richard Blackmore (1650-1729) in *Discourse on Plague,* Part II, said that Wood Sorrel is useful for plague.

Wormwood

Kidney
Nephritis
Taken too often or into large a quantity is irritating to stomach, increases heart action and arteries dangerously
Useful and best in formula
Liver
Jaundice
Fever
Expels worms
Diarrhea
Rheumatism
Swelling
Sprains
William Salmon, *Doron Medicum,* (1644-1713), in Chapter 1, verse 2, says that Wormwood heats, opens obstructions of liver and spleen, and kills worms.

William Salmon in *Family Dictionary* said that that Wormwood is good for yellow jaundice.

Richard Blackmore (1650-1729) in *Discourse on Plague,* Part II, said that Wormwood is good for plague.

B. Frank Scholl, *Library of Health,* 1925 edition:
External applications for ulcers

Samuel Thomson, *New Guide to Health or Botanic Family physician,* 1833:
Stomach
Creates appetite

Yarrow

Hemorrhages
Bleeding from lungs
Fever
Suppressed urine
Mucus in bladder
Douche
Measles
Smallpox
Chickenpox
Piles
Hemorrhage of bowel
Infant diarrhea
Expels gas
Diabetes
Bright's disease
Causes perspiration
Purifies blood
Colds
Flu
Gout
Typhoid fever

Yellow Dock

Tones entire system
Blood purifier

Skin
Glands
Tumors
Swelling
Leprosy
Cancer
Ulcerated eyelids
Syphilis
Runny ears
Swollen glands
High in iron
Ointments

Today medical science reigns supreme and the use of medicinal herbs has become all but a lost art. Now that we have become so frightened about the dangers of using drugs, the hazards of mixing drugs and wrong dosages, people are beginning to place the same concern on the use of herbs. Because of this, people seem to need some instruction as to how much and how to take herbs. One man said, when told about herbs; "do I chew up the plant, make a tea or cook it like cabbage? How much do I take and how do I take it?" The interesting thing about using herbs is that there are no side effects as we find with the use of drugs. When using the mild herbs treated in this book, tried and used experimentally, one will find there are many herbs that will work equally well on one particular disease, and their medicinal uses seem so vast that it would take a lifetime to learn them all. However, there are herbs that grow in every area of the world which seem to relate and work better when one lives in that area in the same way that oranges only grow in given areas under certain climatic circumstances. Crops of any kind are strong or weak depending on soil conditions, the same way that grow in a natural way. Nothing in nature really grows equally. The same goes for people. For a given set of conditions, past and future, through an ever-changing set of circumstances, nature provides a similar kind of plant that will in general do a specific thing when taken into many different kinds of human bodies.

With the production of drugs, we have established a somewhat "closer" scrutiny as to definite chemical analysis, but the dangers of

140

the products themselves have somehow been lost in the shuffle of laboratory testing and scientific research. As long as we know how many terrible things a drug can accomplish, we do not seem to care that it is human life with which we are dealing. Even the most accurate standard of a drug performance seems to be lost on certain people. In attempting to make a perfect equation there always seems to be a variable. It is no different with herbs, as herbs do not cause side effects, but there is a vast difference in the dangers involved. With this in mind the approximates are listed.

Herbs that have been used over the centuries for specific diseases have also been listed. With the recent interest in herbs, manufacturing companies are either putting herbs in powder, capsulating them, forming them into tablets, or making them into tinctures, salves or teas. Because people are turning to the usefulness of herbs as if it were a new idea of a scientific age, the sale of herbs is fast becoming a very lucrative industry. Herbs can be used in any of the above ways. The approximates listed are only guidelines by way of a beginning point. If a person really used herbs in the correct way they would always start out with small amounts and observe how they react. If they do not have the desired result more can be added. Since reactions on mild herbs are never drastic, compared to drugs, it takes time and experimenting with a person's own body to learn which ones work best on a particular body. To learn to live by the spirit within is an all-important factor anytime one embarks on a self-healing program. Call it subconscious, sixth sense, innate intelligence, God, or whatever name you may choose to give it, this then becomes a necessary tool to use in healing the body. When we pay money and rely on a doctor's diagnosis we are only accepting an educated guess, unless he has learned to tap this resource. When we have enough knowledge about a subject to know what to ask, we are then ready to tap into this other realm on her own. It is not my intention to state that there are no doctors who have the ability to tap into this perceptive state on behalf of their patients, but rather to help the reader to recognize that he can find this resource for himself.

If we have concluded, for example, that after fifty some years of drug use and abuse we are in danger from the use of drugs, and if we further learn the herbs that have been known and used with similar results all the way back to the latest written knowledge in the world's existence. With this in mind, healing the body, as by a doctor or by one's self, becomes not only a scientific study but an art. My definition of art is, something creative being brought forth out of an inexplicable concept, somewhere in the resources of consciousness, which sets the artist apart from everyone else who does not know how to be creative. You can either depend on your Doctor and hope he knows how this is done or you can learn for yourself. Anyone who is frightened at this prospect should recognize what has been said, "... that 80% of the time, the body will heal itself in spite of what is done for it, good or bad." Somehow, somewhere, something is on our side, and for a doctor who doesn't know what he is doing those are pretty good odds.

What we do when we learn the rules upon which the body is created, is that after obeying such rules, we tap into this awareness which adds that extra dimension and increases the odds in our behalf. Who is there who is not interested in a healthier, happier existence? In playing the game of life one must learn the rules. One of the major roles which will make the use of herbs more effective and accurate on behalf of healing is to know, first of all, how the body feeds and eliminates. Without this knowledge people have in the past as well as in the present become discouraged with the use of herbs. If the anticipated result of taking herbs is the same as it is with drugs, that the mere taking of a pill will repair all the years of broken health laws, a person will eventually become as disappointed with herbs as they will with drugs. The main laws to learn, then, are that the body heals slowly with herbs and a corrective diet. In serious chronic diseases the diet must be as strict as a semi-fasting, alkaline diet along with the use of cleansing formulas.

It is my opinion that everyone should go on a semi-fast at least a month out of every year and when there is chronic disease, the diet should be continued until all symptoms disappear.

Method for a cleanse: Mild Food Diet

MILD Food in Chronic Sickness	NO Concentrated Foods When Sick
All fruits and vegetables (as much raw as possible)	Grain
	Sugar
Fruit juice (canned, raw, or frozen)	Dairy products
	Butter
Vegetable juice (raw only)	Eggs
Soft oil (raw, cold pressed)	Dried legumes
All nuts (must be raw)	Meat
Honey (raw)	Peanuts
Sprouts (alfalfa, bean, grains)	Chips, etc.
All starch vegetables must be baked – potato, squash, parsnips, yams	

Cleansing Herbs Formulas:

CS
Gentian – 2 parts
Catnip – 1 part
Bayberry bark – 1 part
Goldenseal – 1 part
Myrrh – 1 part
Irish moss – 1 part
Fenugreek seed – 1 part
Chickweed – 1 part
Pink root – 1 part
Comfrey – 1 part

Cyani flowers – ¾ part
Bearfoot root – 1 part
Bugleweed – part
Yellow dock – 1 part
Prickly Ash berries – 1 part
Pulsatilla – 1 part
St. John's wort – 1 part
Blue vervain – 1 part
Mandrake – 1 part
Evening Primrose – 1 part
(Approx. 6 capsules daily; later, lower to 4)

CT FORMULA 1
(where parasites and ulceration of colon are present)
Cayenne – 1 part
Black cohosh – 1 part
Saffron – 1 part
Mandrake - 2 parts
Yellow dock - 2 parts
Blue cohosh - 2 parts
Red clover - 3 parts
Comfrey - 3 parts
Blue vervain - 2 parts
Heal all (parasites) - 2 parts
Nettle (parasites) - 2 parts
Slippery elm - 3 parts

CT FORMULA 2

Gentian - 2 parts
Blue vervain - 1 part
Nettle - 1 part
Red clover - 1 part
Myrrh - 1 part
Mandrake - 2 parts
Bayberry - 1 part
Goldenseal - 1 part
Stillengia - 2 parts
Blue violet - 2 parts
Bearfoot root - 1 part

Bugleweed - 1 part
Yellow dock - 1 part
Prickly ash berries - 1 part
Pulsatilla - 1 part
St. John's wort - 1 part
(Approx. 6 capsules daily; later, lower to 4)

Abscesses

Flaxseed – used as a poultice
Gotu Kola – used as a poultice
Mugwort – used as a poultice
Onion – used as a poultice

Aches

Chamomile tea approximately 4 - 5 cups daily
Chamomile capsules or tablets approximately 4 - 5 daily
Prickly Ash berries approximately 4 capsules daily

Acid stomach

Aspen tea – cups as needed
Catnip tea – cups as needed
Fennel tea – cups as needed
Plantain – approximately 1 capsule as needed
Saffron – approximately 4 to 5 capsules as needed

Acne

Burdock – approximately 1 to 2 capsules daily
Elder tea – approximately 1 cup as needed

Addison's disease

Licorice –1 - 6 capsules daily if on a mild food diet – up to 15
    capsules if on a meat starch diet
Wild Yam – approximately 6 capsules a day

Saffron – approximately 4 - 6 capsules daily – reduces lactic acid buildup – aids digestion

Dandelion reduces acids caused from low adrenal function

After birth pains

Angelica – expels afterbirth – approx. 2 capsules or 2 cups of tea

Fennel – approx. 1 cup tea or 2 capsules – stops after birth pains

Bay leaves tea – helps to expel afterbirth

St. John's wort – stops after birth pains – approx. 2 capsules as needed

Angina Pectoris

Lobelia – approx. 1 capsule as needed – as relaxant

Antibiotic herbs

Goldenseal Root – lung cold or flu – 4 - 5 capsules daily

Antiseptic herbs

Used as a tea – skin wash:
All Heal, White Oak Bark, Plantain, Violet Leaves, Goldenseal Root, Myrrh, Wintergreen

Arthritis

Licorice – approx. 4 - 6 capsules if on mild food diet

Dandelion – approx. 2 - 4 capsules daily

Osteoarthritis

Licorice – approx. 4 - 6 capsules if on mild food diet

Dandelion – approx. 2 - 4 capsules daily

Asthma

Bethroot tea

Black Cohosh tea

Comfrey – approx. 4 - 6 capsules daily
Elecampane – approx. 1 capsule as needed
Licorice as a relaxant – approx. 2 - 4 capsules
Lobelia as a relaxant – approx. 2 - 4 capsules as needed
Hyssop tea – approx. 4 - 5 cups a day
Mullein tea
Nettle tea
Pleurisy root – approx. 1 - 2 capsules or tea
Squaw Vine tea as needed
Vervain acts as a nervine and helps to remove mucus – approx. 2 capsules or 1 cup tea

Bee sting

Nettle poultice or internally as tea – several cups a day

Bladder problems

Alfalfa
All Heal
Bittersweet tea – approx. 1 cup
Chamomile tea
Elecampane – approx. one capsule or 1 cup tea
Marshmallow – approx. 2 capsules or 2 cups tea
Parsley – tea or 3 - 4 tablets
Sassafras – approx. 3 capsules or tea as needed
Slippery Elm – approx. 4 - 6 capsules for bleeding
Goldenseal Root – approx. 3 capsules for bleeding
Squaw Fine – tea as needed
Tansy – tea as needed
Uva Ursi –approx. 4 - 5 cups tea daily
Yarrow – approx. 2 -4 capsules daily or 4 -5 cups tea as needed

Bleeding

Cayenne – approx. 2 - 4 capsules or powdered on wound
Goldenseal root – approx. 2 - 4 capsules for internal bleeding

Breast-feeding

Sage and Parsley – diminishes milk when weaning
Alfalfa increases flow of milk
Red raspberry

Bronchitis

Bayberry – approx. 1 - 2 capsules or tea as needed
Blue Violet tea – 3 - 4 cups a day
Calamus Root 3 - 4 cups a day
Ginger – add 2 other teas
Goldenseal – kills infection – approx. 3 - 4 cups a day
Lemon juice – several times a day
Peach leaves tea – several cups a day or 3 - 4 capsules
Violet tea – approx. 3 -5 cups a day

Chapped hands – skin eruptions

Sarsaparilla – 4 capsules or 4 cups a day

Childbirth

Black cohosh at onset of labor – 2 capsules
Blue cohosh at onset of labor – 2 capsules
Squaw vine 2 months – approx. 2 - 3 capsules daily
Spikenard – approx. one capsule daily the month before delivery;
    approx. 2 capsules 2 weeks before delivery; approx. 3
    capsules the last week
Strawberry and Raspberry – approx. 2 -3 capsules daily through
    entire 9 months

Colds

Alfalfa tea – 6 cups per day
Aspen tea – for pain – 2 cups as needed
Bay leaves tea
Blue Violet tea (produces perspiration taken hot)

Chamomile tea

Cayenne – 4 - 5 capsules a day

Catnip – as relaxant for pain (produces perspiration taken hot)

Elder tea from flowers – for glandular swelling

Fenugreek – for fever – 2 capsules or 2 cups tea

Juniper – activates kidneys, relieves pain – 2 capsules or as needed

Lemon juice and honey – drink throughout the day

Mullein tea – for glandular swelling and difficult breathing – or 2 to 3 capsules

Nettle – kills parasites, activates kidneys, relieves shortness of breath, helps to expel mucus, helps headache – 1 - 2 capsules as needed

Red Clover – relieves hard breathing – relaxant

Sarsaparilla tea as needed

Tansy – 2 - 4 capsules (increases urine flow)

Valerian – relaxant, promotes sleep, relieves pain, – 2 capsules as needed

Vervain – produces perspiration, helps breathing, overcomes coughing

Wood Betony – for pain and headache – 2 capsules

Yarrow tea

Colitis

Black Walnut – kills worms – 2 - 4 capsules

Slippery Elm – 4 - 6 capsules

Goldenseal root – 2 capsules

Psyllium – 1 - 2 tablespoons in water per day

Licorice – 2 - 4 capsules a day

Diarrhea

Bayberry tea – 1 quart tea to 1 quart water – used in enema

Psyllium – 1 - 2 tablespoons in water or juice per day

Slippery Elm

Infant diarrhea

Yarrow tea
Carob powder mixed in milk

Digestion

Barberry – 1 cup tea or one capsule
Psyllium – 1 - 2 tablespoons in water per day
Bungle weed – approx. 1 capsule
Cascara Sagrada is helpful to digestion, but is a laxative – any
    laxative amount would improve digestion
Dandelion – approx. 1 - 2 capsules
Ginseng – approx. 3 - 4 capsules daily
Peppermint tea as needed
Red raspberry – approx. 1 - 3 capsules
Spearmint tea – 1 cup as needed
All condiment herbs have an influence on digestion

Diphtheria

Bay leaves tea – approx. 6 cups daily
Myrrh – approx. 2 capsules twice daily

Dizziness

Peppermint tea – as needed
Plain water enema – for fluid build up
Dandelion tea – as needed
Goldenseal root – approx. 4 - 5 capsules daily

Dysentery

Bay enema
Gentian – approx. 3 capsules daily
Marshmallow – approx. 6 capsules daily
Peppermint tea – as needed
Plantain – approx. 3 capsules daily
Saffron – approx. 4 - 6 capsules daily
Uva Ursi – approx. 2 - 4 capsules daily

Ears

Cleavers drops in ears for pain
Eyebright – approx. 2 capsules – for earache
Hops
Mullein – approx. 3 to 4 caps daily
Mullein tincture for fungus – 2 - 4 drops as needed
Wood Betony – approx. 2 capsules for pain

Eczema

Burdock – blood cleanser – approx. 3 - 4 capsules daily
Dandelion – reduces uric acid – approx. 3 - 4 capsules daily
Poke Root – cleans lymph retention – approx. 1 - 2 capsules
    daily
Flaxseed poultice – cook with water until thick – apply

Edema

Hyssop tea – drink approx. 6 - 8 cups daily
Tansy tea – fluid build up

Epilepsy

Betony
Blue Cohosh – approx. 1 capsule as needed
Catnip – approx. 1 - 2 capsules for relaxant
Hops – approx. 1 - 2 capsules as needed for relaxant
Lady Slipper – approx. 4 capsules as needed for relaxant
Lobelia – approx. 1 capsule
Skullcap – approx. 2 capsules
Valerian – approx. 2 capsules
Vervain – approx. 2 - 4 capsules

Eyes

Chickweed tea – wash for sore eyes – make tea, strain, and use
    eye cup or dropper
Elder – twitching eyelid

Eyebright – internally and as eye wash with Goldenseal root
Mallow – wash for sore eyes
Plantain – internally and wash – approx. 1 - 2 capsules
Rosemary – strengthens eyes – approx. 1 - 2 capsules
Sassafras – wash for inflamed eyes
Squaw vine – wash for sore eyes

Female organs

Dandelion – overcomes acidity – approx. 2 - 4 capsules daily
Gentian – approx. 2 - 3 capsules
Black Cohosh – approx. 1 - 2 capsules
Ginger – for menstrual cramps – approx. 3 - 4 capsules

Fever

Cayenne – approx. 1- 2 capsules every 3 hours
Goldenseal root – antibiotic – approx. 4 - 5 capsules daily
To activate kidneys:
   Alfalfa tea
   Uva Ursi tea
   Cornsilk tea
   Juniper tea
   Dandelion tea
   Watermelon seed tea
Hot saffron tea – causes perspiration
Violet tea causes perspiration

Gallbladder

See - *Is Any Sick Among You?* for the gallstone purge.
Dandelion – approx. 2 capsules daily
Lemon juice
Saffron – approx. 4 - 6 capsules daily (flushes gallbladder)
Fennel – approx. 2 - 3 capsules daily

Gout

All Heal – approx. 4 capsules daily

Blue Violet tea – causes perspiration, overcomes acid through skin

Dandelion – overcomes uric acid – approx. 3 capsules with every meal containing meat, otherwise 4 daily

Ginger

Headache

Enema for any headache

Aspen Bark tea as needed

Betony – approx. 1 capsule as needed

Catnip – for nervous headache – approx. 2 - 4 capsules

Eyebright – approx. 2 - 4 capsules

Fennel – approx. 1 - 3 capsules

Senna – approx. 1 capsule as laxative

Peppermint tea

Nettle tea

Peach Bark tea

Rosemary tea

Squaw vine tea (Brigham tea)

Vervain – approx. 2 - 4 capsules – for nervous headache

Violet tea

Wood Betony – for pain

Formula – equal parts: Peppermint, Marjoram, Thyme, Rosemary – 2 - 3 capsules or tea as needed

Infection

Goldenseal root – approx. 1 - 5 capsules daily

Bayberry – approx. 2 - 4 capsules daily

Echinacea – approx. 1 - 2 capsules

Cayenne – approx. 2 - 3 capsules as needed

Influenza

Peppermint tea

Alfalfa tea

Catnip tea

Goldenseal root – approx. 1 - 5 capsules daily
Lemon and honey – no added water – tablespoon hourly
Wood Betony – for pain – 1 as needed
Aspen Bark tea – approx. 1 cup as needed for pain

Insect bite

Bay leaf tea – as wash
Goldenseal root – antibiotic – approx. 2 - 4 capsules
Borage tea – as wash
Fennel – as wash or poultice
Juniper oil – apply to bite
Parsley tea – as wash

Kidneys

Agrimony tea
Alfalfa tea or approx. 6 - 8 capsules
All Heal – approx. 2 capsules
Barberry – best used in a formula
Bethroot tea
Bitterroot tea
Buchu tea – especially helpful in prostate problems
Chamomile tea or – approx. 2 - 3 capsules
Cayenne – preferably in a formula
Comfrey – ulceration of kidneys
Dandelion – approx. 2 - 4 capsules daily – increases flow of
    urine
Elder bark tea – for water retention from kidneys or heart
Flaxseed tea – for inflammation of kidneys – approx. 2 - 4 cups
Horsetail – tea as needed – excellent as diuretic – or approx. 1 - 3
    capsules as needed
Hyssop tea – approx. 6 cups a day
Mallow – approx. 1 - 3 capsules a day
Marshmallow – approx. 4 capsules a day
Parsley – tea as needed – or approx. 4 - 6 tablets or capsules a
    day
Pleurisy root tea
Poke Root – best used in formula

154

Poplar tea
Queen of the meadow – approx. 1 - 4 capsules or tablets
Sage tea
Sanicle tea
Sassafras – approx. 2 - 4 capsules
Tansy – approx. 2 - 3 capsules
Wood Betony – kidney obstructions
Asparagus and Celery are excellent vegetables for kidneys

Liver obstructions

Agrimony – jaundice and obstructions – approx. 1 capsule every 4 hours
All Heal – approx. 1 - 2 caps every 4 hours
Angelica tea – 4 - 5 cups daily
Goldenseal root – for cleansing liver – approx. 1 - 2 capsules as needed
Raw Beet juice– excellent for cleaning liver
Lemon and Water – excellent for cleaning liver
Saffron –approx. 2 - 4 capsules a day – when taken hot in tea causes perspiration

Lungs

Lung formula:
   Mullein – 1 part
   Comfrey – 1 part
   Marshmallow – 1 part
   Slippery Elm – 1 part
   Lobelia – 1/2 part
Approx. 2 - 4 capsules as needed

Morning sickness

Peach leaves – approx. 2 capsules as needed
Goldenseal root – approx. 1 - 2 capsules as needed
Saffron – approx. 1 - 2 capsules as needed
Dandelion – approx. 1 - 2 capsules as needed
Peppermint tea – as needed

Muscular pains

Chamomile tea – approx. 4 - 6 cups daily
Wood Betony – approx. 1 capsule as needed
Aspen Bark – approx. 1 capsule as needed
Dandelion – approx. 1 - 2 capsules as needed

Nervousness

Sarsaparilla tea as needed
Valerian – approx. 2 - 3 capsules as needed
Skullcap – approx. 2 capsules as needed
Hops – approx. 2 capsules as needed – see formula section
Lady slipper – approx. 2 - 4 capsules – especially helpful when caused by brain damage
Gotu-Kola – approx. 2 - 3 as needed for nervous breakdown
Vervain – approx. 1 - 2 capsules as needed

Pain

Wood Betony – approx. 2 - 4 capsules as needed
Aspen – approx. 2 - 4 capsules as needed
Valerian – approx. 2 - 3 capsules as needed to relax nerves
Pleurisy root tea – 1 cup as needed
Lobelia – approx. 1 - 3 capsules as needed
Hops – approx. 1 - 2 capsules as needed or tea

Pyorrhea

Cayenne – approx. 2 capsules
Goldenseal – approx. 2 - 3 capsules a day – is also as mouthwash
Myrrh – used as mouthwash

Rheumatic fever

Pleurisy Root – approx. 2 - 4 capsules daily
Sarsaparilla tea – approx. 4 - cups or 4 capsules daily
Squaw vine – tea as needed

Rheumatism

Aspen tea – for pain
Black Cohosh – approx. 1 capsule
Blue Cohosh – approx. 1 capsule
Burdock – approx. 2 - 4 capsules daily – blood purifier
Cayenne – 1 capsule with each meal
Chickweed – approx. 2 capsules as needed
Dandelion – approx. 2 capsules with each meal
Gotu-Kola
Horse radish – raw used in salad or salad dressing

Scalds

Elder – use leaves in poultice
Nettle – as poultice
Plantain – as poultice
Aloe vera – cut leaf and use gel right on burn
Comfrey – crush leaves – uses poultice

Sciatica

Aspen – 1 cup as needed for pain
Juniper – approx. 1 - 2 capsules
St. John's wort – approx. 1 - 2 capsules

Sexual glands

Fo-ti-tieng – approx. 1 - 3 capsules or as tea
Hops – approx. 1 - 2 capsules or tea as needed for relaxant
Mexican Damiana – approx. 1 - 2 capsules – only as relaxant
Skullcap – approx. 1 - 3 capsules

Shock

Catnip – approx. 2 - 4 capsules
Hops – approx. 2 - 4 capsules
Lady slipper – approx. 3 -4 capsules
Lobelia – approx. 1 capsule as needed

Peppermint tea – make strong and sip continuously
Valerian – approx. 1 -3 capsules

Sleep

Catnip – approx. 1 - 4 capsules
Hops – approx. 1 - 4 capsules
Lady slipper – approx. 1 - 4 capsules
Skullcap – approx. 1 - 3 capsules
Valerian – approx. 1 - 3 capsules

Sore throat

Bayberry tea – several cups as needed – also good as gargle
Black Walnut – approx. 1 - 3 capsules daily
Blue Violet – causes perspiration
Echinacea – approx. 1 - 2 capsules
Elderberries – fresh juice is good as a laxative and a gargle
Ginger tea
Horehound made into a candy with honey
Lemon juice – as gargle or with honey
Myrrh – as a gargle
Nettle tea

Sores

Aloes – as poultice
Blue Violet – made into a tea and used as a skin wash
Chamomile – for skin wash
Chickweed tea – for skin wash
Comfrey – bruise leaves and use as a poultice
Dandelion tea – as a wash
Goldenseal root tea – as a skin wash or use dry powder on open
    wound
Peach leaves – poultice
Queen of the meadow tea – as wash

Stomach

Bayberry tea – or approx. one capsule
Comfrey – approx. 2 - 3 capsules
Fennel tea
Flaxseed – made into a thick tea
Ginseng – approx. 1 - 2 capsules
Goldenseal root – approx. 1 - 2 capsules
Hops – tea or capsules – relaxant for nervous stomach
Marjoram – condiment used in cooking helps digestion
Nettle tea
Peach tea – or approx. 1 - 2 capsules
Dandelion – approx. 2 - 4 capsules
Saffron – approx. 2 - 4 capsules
Sassafras tea
Slippery Elm – approx. 1 - 4 capsules for ulcers
Spearmint tea – 1 cup as needed
White Willow tea
Wood Betony – approx. 1 capsule as needed for pain

Tonsils

Burdock – approx. 1 - 3 capsules or tea throughout the day
Echinacea – approx. 1 capsule 4 times daily – for swelling in the throat
Mullein – approx. 1 capsule 4 times a day

Toothache

All Heal – approx. 2 - 4 capsules
Angelica – approx. 2 - 4 capsules
Oil of Clove on tooth with cotton
Hops – approx. 2 - 4 capsules for pain
Marjoram – as tea
Oil of Peppermint on tooth and gum with cotton
Prickly ash bark – as tea

Tuberculosis

Burdock – approx. as many as 5 capsules a day
comfrey – approx. 6 capsules a day or tea

Mullein – approx. 4 - throughout the day
Nettle – as tea

Typhoid fever

Bay leaves – as tea
Bittersweet – as tea
Chamomile – as tea
Goldenseal root – approx. 4 - 6 capsules a day
Myrrh – as gargle
Pleurisy root – as tea
Yarrow – as tea or capsules for a day
Lemon – straight to dissolve the membrane that develops in the
   throat

Ulcers

Bethroot – approx. 2 - 3 capsules 20 minutes before eating
Blue Violet – as tea
Cayenne – approx. 4 - X capsules
Chickweed – approx. 1 capsule before meal
Dandelion – approx. 2 to 3 capsules as needed – reduces acidity
   of stomach
Flaxseed – make thick tea and drink cup as needed
Goldenseal root – approx. 1 capsule before meal when infection
   and inflammation are involved – antibiotic
Hops tea – for nervous stomach
Horsetail tea – reduces acidity
Mullein – approx. 1 - 2 capsules before meal
Slippery Elm – approx. 2 - 3 capsules 20 minutes before meal
Wood Betony – approx. 1 capsule for pain as needed

Vomiting

Colombo tea – stops vomiting
Red Raspberry tea – stops vomiting
Lobelia – approx. 2 - 3 capsules or more to produce vomiting –
   use with strong peppermint tea

Virgil J. Vogel, in his book *American Indian Medicine*, has done a wonderful research, with many pages of bibliography, much of it unpublished. It is very well done and could be a start for anyone interested in a study of American and Indian historical medicine.

He writes about Doctor Samuel Thomson, whom I mentioned in my book, *Is Any Sick Among You?*, Being connected to the life of Willard Richards and is also discussed in Jethro Kloss' his book, *Back to Eden*.

According to the books I have read, Doctor Samuel Thomson achieved a great deal of fame in his field before being attacked by certain medical doctors, causing him much expense and heart ache. His important discovery was Lobelia, and because it was such a powerful emetic, he had difficulty convincing many people of its value.

On page 4 regarding yellow fever he said that "those who had regular positions died."

> *"The word quackery, when used against me, was a very important charm to prejudice the people against my practice: but I would ask all the candid and reflecting past of the people, the following question, and I will leave them to their conscience to give an answer: which is the greatest quack, the one who relieves them from their sickness by the most simple and safe means, without any pretense to infallibility skill, more than what nature and experience had taught him, or the one who, instead of curing the disease, increases it by distress of the patient, till either the strength of his natural constitution or death relieves him?"*

On page 58 he said:

"The Doctor was paid a heavy bill for his visits; but my cure was done so quick that it was thought not to be worthy of their notice, and I never received a cent from them for my trouble."

Doctor Thomson was called upon to care for a child. After treating her he left with the usual agreement to return the next day. In the meantime, another Doctor was called in on the case who said Doctor Thomson's method (the natural Herb method) would not work so Doctor Thomson was removed from the case. Doctor Thomson said of the other Doctor:

"He filled it with Mercury and ran it down: after having given as much Mercury inside as nature could move, and the bowels grew silent, he then rubbed mercurial ointment on the bowel as long as it had any effect; after which he agreed that the child had the canker very badly but he still persisted in the same course till the child was wasted away and died in about two months after it was 1st taken sick. After the child was dead, it's parents were willing to allow that I understood the disorder best. The Doctor got $20 for killing the child by inches and I got nothing."

Doctor Samuel Thomson's life was filled with many hardships, both as a child and as an adult. Because of an analytical, scientific mind, coupled with the same spirituality I have observed in the other physicians of the past, he seemed to quickly and easily draw a correct conclusion. He could see how by natural herbal methods and correct laws marvelous results could be achieved. He was at a loss to understand how medical doctors of his day could maintain their integrity with such pretensions as they made, dabbling at the art of healing. Despite heavy pressures from the growing established medical practices of his time, he continued to help whenever he could, always confident that his best tool was truth. He was an uneducated man as to accredited schooling. His education had been practical from a childhood knowledge of the use of and handling of herbs on into adult practice helping and serving the sick. He seemed to be compelled by the knowledge he possessed to continue to serve mankind regardless of the consequences to himself. His aim was apparently worthy of the sacrifice of his individual advantage.

Who's Who in America says of him:

"He had many court trials because of his methods of healing. This seems to be the only thing remembered about him."

As I read his narrative of his own life, I see such a parallel today with the many naturopathics who have been so persecuted for their knowledge of the truth. Such a lonely ordeal they have faced because they have touched the most sensitive nerve, which today causes us to be trapped into chemical therapy (big money). Understanding how the body feeds and eliminates would cause us to recognize that elimination is not a side effect at all but rather nature's way to rid us of those elements causing pain or obstruction in the body. Some herbs are more laxative than others, so if it were understood to let nature, along with the herbs, slowly remove obstruction, we would all have the good sense not to take too much that is highly laxative and move waste faster than the body's ability to rebuild or throw it out.

Many are beginning to abandon this long, almost ideological, tradition of modern medicine and return to nature for the answers. Many have reached a turning point and are overcoming the mental stagnation caused by men who care about nothing but how much money they can make off the misfortunes of their fellowmen. Intelligent people everywhere are beginning to feel a wave of pure joy sweep over them as they recognize these truths – new to them in all their grand simplicity. With this understanding, they refused to be compelled by events of our time to pay the high cost of death.

When we come to believe and understand a correct principle, our feelings about this knowledge become very intense and with a concentrated effort, we desire to live by these principles even at the risk of sacrifice.

The battle between truth and error is always culminated into the fruits of bitter contest, causing among those who did not take sides to be left in panic and uncertainty. As the medical chemicals lose their stranglehold upon the people and the almost godlike prestige of the doctor fades from world consciousness, we could see a gravely presented spectacle of general fear among those who have no idea how to look to the resources about them, let alone how to look within their souls or to tap the heavenly realm by prayer. We have too long leaned upon the arm of flesh and it has, as Jeremiah said, been a curse to us.

A change could erupt with extraordinary suddenness as the economy becomes worse with prices reaching unprecedented heights. The first thing to be laid by the wayside would be insurance, followed by the high medical cash costs, and man could again luckily be left to his own cunning and resourcefulness. There is little doubt he would then be forced to give serious consideration to a less sophisticated idea of how to take care of his health. He may find, to his utter amazement, that all this complicated medical science he had been brainwashed into believing, was a farce which had not the capacity to endure when people are forced to stand up on their own feet. When we understand the simplicity of truth, we develop a quiet confidence and a prayerful gratitude for knowledge shared with a wise and great God.

Doctor Thomson said that Lobelia is a emetic but not cathartic.

"This plant is different in one very important particular, from all others that I have knowledge of, that is the same quantity will produce the same effect in all stages of its growth, from its first appearance till it comes to maturity."

He said with the use of Lobelia:

"I have seen some lie and sob like a child that has been punished for two hours, not able to speak or raise

their hands, to use their head and the next day be about and soon get well.

"In cases where they have taken considerable opium and this medicine (Lobelia) is administered, it will in its operation, produce the same appearance and symptoms that are produced by opium when first given, which having lain dormant, is roused into action by the enlivening qualities of this medicine and the patient will often be thrown into a senseless state: the whole system will be one complete massive confusion, tumbling in every direction, and it will take 2 or 3 to hold them on the bed. The times they grow cold as though dying; remaining in this way from 2 to 8 hours, and then awake, like one from sleep, after a good night's rest, entirely calm and sensible as though nothing ailed them. It is seldom they ever have more than one of these turns; as it is the last struggle of the disease and they gradually begin to recover from that time."

This could be an answer to drug abuse. It could be an interesting research project. He claims in all the many years of his practice, he used this Herb and cayenne on all kinds of disease with favorable results.

Thomson said:

"Avoid all minerals used as medicine, such as mercury, arsenic, antinomy, calomel, preparations of copper or lead; also nitre and opium. They are all deadly poisons and enemies of health."

Priddy Meeks, who was mentioned also in my book *Is Any Sick Among You?* as being with Willard Richards, a part of the 1st medical society of Utah. Quoting from his Journal writings, he said regarding the use of Lobelia, page 46:

"Lobelia will act on the system in complete conformity with the laws of health, and when that law is obstructed and fails to fulfill the operations that nature intended it to fulfill while healthy, it will remove those obstructions

165

wherever located. For Lobelia will permeate the whole system until it finds where the obstruction is seated, and there it will spend its influence and powers by relaxing the parts obstructed. There should always accompany the Lobelia with cayenne pepper, which is the purest and best stimulant that is known in the compass of medicine. It will increase the very life and vitality of the system and give the blood a greater velocity and power. Now the system being so relaxed with Lobelia and the blood being so stimulated with such power, it will act on the whole system. It will act on the whole system like an increased flow of water turned into a muddy spring of water – it will soon run clear. And although Lobelia is set anought and persecuted the way it is, it is for the same reason that the latter-day Saints are persecuted. It is ordained of God to be used in wisdom. The world will not persecute them that are like them. It is stated that Joseph Smith said that Thomson was as much inspired to bring forth his principle of practice according to the dignity and importance of it as an appendix to the gospel as a temporal salvation. It was introduced nearly contemporary with the Gospel, even the Word of Wisdom and Thomsonianism runs together and strengthens each other, instead of coming in collision with each other. Thomson was uneducated the same as Joseph Smith was. He had not much experience the same as Joseph Smith and was not of high parentage, so thought by the world the same as Joseph Smith was. They tried to kill him the same as they did Joseph Smith. They lanced him the same as they did Joseph Smith, and did everything in their power to stop its progress, but could not do it, because it was inspiration and, of course, of Divine origin like Joseph Smith's mission, and has never lacked opposition ever since it was introduced, just like Mormonism, and that is one evidence of its being correct. For the prophets have said, there must needs be an opposition in all things, and they have also said it must need be that offenses come, but woe unto them by whom they come."

On page 29 he said:

"I sometimes look upon Lobelia as being supernatural, although I have been using it for (46) years. I do not know the extent of its powers and virtues in restoring the sick and at the same time perfectly harmless. It is undoubtedly the best and purest relaxum in the compass of medicine. That is the reason it is so good in childbed cases. It puts the system exactly in the situation the laws of nature would have it be to perform that object. Those in the habit of using it in such cases look forward in pleasing application of having a good time without the forebodings of trouble so common to women. Oh! glorious medicine!"

He says *"Oh! glorious medicine!"* Many times in his Journal with such gratitude for so wonderful a cure.

Some Formulas – Home Remedies

The formulas listed below are some of the most popular. Many or most of these formulas are put together by Herb manufacturers and can often be found in Herb shops, Health food stores and Direct Sales persons. However, we are not permitted to mention any specific company.

We have written the approximate number of capsules or tablets that can be used. But this varies for each individual and their particular need at the time.

Arthritic Formula
(Approx.4 - 6 daily)
Yucca
Licorice
Alfalfa
Chaparral
Yarrow
Cayenne
Dandelion
Centaury
Burdock Root

Cascara Sagrada

Asthma formula
(Approx.2 - as needed)
Blessed Thistle
Black Cohosh
Skull Cap
Pleurisy Root
Licorice

Athletic Formula

(Approx.6 cups daily or as needed)
Saffron
Dandelion
Gentian
Skullcap
Valerian
Buckthorn Bush
Cayenne
Wild Yam

Cleansing Formula

(Approx.4 - 6 daily)
Gentian
Catnip
Golden Seal
Barberry Bark
Myrrh
Comfrey
Yellow Dock
Fenugreek
Bugleweed
Irish Moss
Pink Root
Cyani Flowers
Mandrake
Chickweed
Black Walnut
Dandelion
St. John's wort
Echinacea

Cold Formula

(Approx.3 every 4 hrs.)
Rose Hips
Chamomile
Slippery Elm
Yarrow

Goldenseal Root
Peppermint
Cayenne
Lemon Grass
Sage
Myrrh
Senna

Ear Infection

(Approx.2 every 3 hours)
Echinacea
Golden Seal Root
Poke Root
Capsicum

Energy Formula

(Approx.3 daily)
Gotu Kola
Ginseng
Capsicum

Eye Wash Formula

(Cataracts: Use eye cup, dissolve powder in warm water; strain through cloth towel)
Eyebright
Goldenseal Root
Bayberry

Female Formula

(Approx.4 daily)
Red Clover
Goldenseal Root
Parsley
Queen of the Meadow
Blessed Thistle
Marshmallow

Lobelia
Ginger
Black Cohosh
Red Raspberry
Squaw Vine

Gastritis Formula
(Approx. 2 -3 as needed)
Equal parts:
  Slippery Elm
  Raspberry Leaves
Half part:
  Marshmallow
  Agrimony

Headache Formula
(Approx. 2 or more as needed)
Equal parts:
  Peppermint
  Marjoram
  Thyme
  Rosemary

Heart Combination
(Approx. 3 - 4 daily)
Hawthorne Berries
Capsicum
Garlic

High Blood Pressure
(Approx. 2-4 as needed)
(Where there is cholesterol; not for high blood pressure or hyper-tension type)
Capsicum
Garlic

Indigestion Formula
(Approx. 1-2 as needed)
Equal parts:
  Centaury
  Agrimony
  Columbo Root
Half part:
  Raspberry Leaves
  Bayberry Bark
Equal parts:
  Centaury
  Raspberry Leaves
  Cleavers
  Dandelion

Infection – Hypoglycemic Formula
(for those who cannot use goldenseal root)
(Approx. 2 - 4 as needed every - 4 hours)
Echinacea
Myrrh Gum
Yarrow
Capsicum

Kidney Formula No. 1
(Approx. 1 - 3 as needed)
Equal parts:
  Asparagus root
  Parsley root
  Celery root
  Fennel

Kidney Formula No. 2
(Approx. 2 - 4 as needed)
Uva Ursi
Parsley
Dandelion

Juniper berries
Sassafras
Chamomile

Laxative formula
(Approx. 1 - 2 as needed)
One part:
  Mandrake
Fourth part:
  Cayenne
  Myrrh Gum

Liver Formula
(Approx. 2
Equal parts:
  Yarrow
  Barberry
  Centaury
  Dandelion
Lobelia
One part:
  Mandrake
  Dandelion
  Gentian
Half part:
  Cleavers
  Goldenseal root
Quarter Part:
  Cayenne

Lung Formula
(Approx. 2 - 3 as needed)
Mullein
Comfrey
Marshmallow
Slippery Elm
Lobelia

Persistent Lung & Bronchial Infections:
(Approx. 2 - 3 as needed; 4 - 6 hours apart)
Lady Slipper
Slippery Elm
Comfrey
Alfalfa
Mullein
Marshmallow
Lobelia
Cayenne
Licorice
Poke Root
Mandrake

Mucus in the Lungs Formula
(Approx. 2 -4 daily)
    Thyme
Fenugreek

Muscles – Muscular Dystrophy Formula
(Approx. 6 - 8 daily)
Vitamin B_1
Vitamin B_2
Biotin
Niacin
Pantothenic Acid
Vitamin E
Calcium
Magnesium
Phosphorus
Potassium
Copper
Manganese
Kelp
Mullein
Alfalfa

Parsley
Raspberry
Licorice
Burdock Root
Yellow Dock
Mandrake
Comfrey
Lady slipper

Nephritis Formula

(Approx. 2 -6 daily)
Equal parts:
  Marshmallow
  Uva Ursi
  Cleavers (leaves)
  Juniper Berries
  Buchu
  Slippery Elm

Nervous Headache Formula

(Approx. 2 as needed)
Equal parts:
  Wood Betony
  Rosemary
  Peppermint

Nervous Tension Formula

(Approx. 2 - 4 as needed)
Lobelia
Valerian
Black cohosh
Mistletoe
Hops
St. John's wort
Wood Betony

Nerve Tonic

(Approx. 2 - 4 as needed
Equal parts:

Skullcap
Hops
Gentian Root
Valerian Root

Obesity Formula

(Approx. 6 - 8 daily)
Five parts:
  Chickweed (dissolves fat)
Two parts:
  Licorice (adrenal hormone)
  Saffron (uric acid buildup)
  Gotu Kola (general cleanse)
  Mandrake (laxative)
  Echinacea (glands)
  Black Walnut (kills
parasites)
One part:
  Hawthorne (heart: edema)
One-half part:
  Fennel (kills appetite)
Also:
  Papaya
  Dandelion

Pain Formula No. 1

(Approx. 1 -3 as needed)
Equal parts:
  Wild Lettuce
  Hops
  Valerian
  Catnip
One-fourth part:
  Lobelia

Pain Formula No. 2

(Approx. 2 - 4 as needed)
Valerian
Wild lettuce

Capsicum
St. John's wort

Parasite Formula
(Approx. 6 daily)
Equal parts:
  Papaya
  Wormwood
  Worm seed
  Pomegranate Root
  Tansy
  Walnut
  Wild Sage
  Tame Sage
  Garlic Powder
One-half part:
  Fennel seed
One-fourth part:
  Senna
(Approx. 1/2 teaspoon powder
morning and night.)
(This formula is useful for all
types of parasites, including
cancer.)

**Parasite Herbal Pumpkin
Formula**
(Approx. 4 - 6 daily)
Pumpkin seed
Culver Root
Mandrake
Violet Leaves
Poke Root
Cascara Sagrada
Which Hazel
Mullein
Comfrey Root
Slippery Elm

Poultice Formula
Comfrey
Goldenseal Root
Slippery Elm
Aloe Vera

Prostate Formula
(Approx. 4 - 6 daily)
Pumpkin Seed
Kelp
Gotu Kola
Licorice
Lobelia
Ginger
Goldenseal Root
Ginseng
Buchu
Yarrow
Senna

Respiratory Condition Formula
(Approx. 3 - 4 as needed)
Comfrey
Fenugreek

Sexual Debility Formula
(Approx. 2 - 4 daily)
Equal parts:
  Gotu Kola
  Saw Palmetto
  Ginseng

Sleep Formula
(Approx. 2 - 4 as needed)
Valerian
Skullcap
Hops

Stomach and Liver Formula

(Approx. 2 as needed)
Equal parts:
  Barberry
  Agrimony
  Centaury
  Meadowsweet

Ulcer Formula
(Approx. 2 - 3 before meals)
Goldenseal Root
Capsicum
Myrrh Gum
Slippery Elm

Urinary Tract
(Approx. 2 - 4 as needed)
Kelp
Black Cohosh
Hydrocotyle Asiatica
Licorice
Goldenseal Root
Lobelia
Capsicum
Ginger
Capsicum

Thyroid Formula
(Approx. 3 - 6 as needed)
Irish Moss
Kelp
Parsley

CHAPTER 4

ART OF RELAXATION
MAKE PEACE WITH YOURSELF
BE OF GOOD CHEER

The Art of Relaxation

A number of years ago I learned from a book on eye exercise a most wonderful way to relax. Because there is so much tension or what is called stress today, if we are to be well, it is important to know how to turn off our problems and relax. We have developed our civilization to such a racing pace that to slow down even causes feelings of guilt barring our escape to repentance. If we are to find the doorway to repentance, which is the beginning of peace, we must have time to think and reflect on past mistakes. We must have time to remember past pleasures, that our hearts may be filled with gratitude. My father used to say the greatest sin was the sin of ingratitude.

Doctrine & Covenants 78:17-19

"Verily, verily, I say unto you, ye are little children, and ye have not as yet understood how great blessings the Father hath in his own hands and prepared for you;

"And ye cannot bear all things now; nevertheless, be of good cheer, for I will lead you along. The kingdom is yours and the blessings thereof are yours, and the riches of eternity are yours.

"And he who receiveth all things with thankfulness shall be made glorious; and the things of this earth shall be added unto him, even an hundred fold, yea, more."

How can we begin to express gratitude when this driving force of fast-moving society with growing complexity fastens us to a treadmill? Every new day is a looming shadow and every yesterday was filled with fatigue, conflict, and a profound anguish. Somewhere along this road we must take time out to enjoy life, to think, to create something lovely, to listen to beautiful music, to learn something beautiful, to do something nice for someone. We become so concerned with economic strength and with financial security that life finally serves no useful purpose but to exist.

J.M. Gibby said:

"Security is not born of inexhaustible wealth but of unquenchable faith."

After living at such a pace, jubilation is short-lived with only a wave of joy sweeping across us now and then. "Man is that he might have joy," but how it eludes us when life becomes such a lonely ordeal.

When a certain man was asked why he had gotten rid of his nagging, hateful wife after the 40 some years he had lived with her wretchedness, he said, "Well, she will be different in the next world." It is sad that this man does not understand that this life is but a brief episode in the great expense of eternity, and we will always be ourselves. Today is the time to create a turning point in our personality, and we are the only ones who can do it. Tomorrow and yesterday are still a part of eternity. We have always existed, there never was a time when we were not, and no one can really imagine such a time, when they stop to think about it.

Did you ever think as you looked at the television shows about a time machine that you would like to step back into time in your full flesh and blood form and live with different people of history? I do not believe in reincarnation. That would seem such a nightmare. This brief life is long enough to have the veil drawn across our remembrance of eternity's past. We do go back, however, in books, and we relive moments in our life by the wonderful memory computer built into our brain. How many times has it seemed sad to you as you have watched your children grow up, that you have lost that adorable little baby to a different, full-grown form and sometimes into a person you hardly know? Did you ever think how fun it would be to go back into time and hold that baby or young child in your arms and feel the kiss of sweet smelling flesh against your lips and feel once more the joy of loving someone so unselfishly, and deeply? Did you ever stop to think at the end of a weary day as you bent over a little bed and kissed the matted hair and perspiring forehead of a tiny little soul you love so much, "Where has the day gone, and I have hardly spent any time with this little one?" "Today is gone and tomorrow he will be bigger, and there is no way I can bring back this day."

There is a way we can bring back a beautiful day, but the day must have existed. To accomplish the exercise I'm going to teach you will take concentrated effort at first then it will begin to be a natural part of your peaceful moments.

First of all, make a quiet place or time when you can be alone. Sit with your hands in a cupping shape over your eyes. Place your elbows in a comfortable place. If you see a lot of lights and colors, you are in a very nervous state. When you get to a point where there is nothing but black with no color, you will have become completely relaxed. Now, I will show you the way to bring about a state of relaxation. Choose a sweet memory of the past from a time when you were completely relaxed, the moments or things that caused you to relax. As you begin to think about it, think it through from beginning to end in every detail from odors, to sounds, to voices, to physical feelings you had, such as touch, joy, peace, relaxation.

To give you an example, I will go through an experience which helps me to relax. Because I relax better laying in the sun than almost any other way I can think of, we will travel together through my pleasant sun bath.

My thoughts returned the beginning of an adventure I have lived many times. The pattern was similar each time, so I will proceed as I walk on to the sandy steps leading from the pier at Santa Cruz to the beach below. As I step onto the steep stairs and hold onto the handrail, maneuvering all the paraphernalia necessary for a sun bath at the beach, I have a feeling of warmth on my body. The sand feels lumpy under my sandaled feet on the hard surface of the stairs. I survey the scene below with the feeling of exhilaration and delight at the prospect of a peaceful day at the beach. The sky is a deep blue and the lagoon is quiet, the surf almost like it belongs on a mountain lake. The pungent smell of the ocean and the damp salt air seem to caress my body, a feeling of nostalgia sweeps momentarily over my mind as I remember all the past good times that accompanied a day at the beach. When my feet touch the beach and I proceed to a place to settle in for a few hours, my unprotected feet, except for the barefoot sandals feel hot as the hurried struggle through deep, warm sand begins, and I remember the feeling of sand flipping from my sandals, hot on the back of my bare legs. Moving closer to the wet, cool sand at the water's edge, I suddenly feel one with the surf, the air, the sky, and the gulls who dip down past me with their familiar cry. Even the people on the beach, the cars moving above on the pier, the hustle and bustle of the fish stores, the restaurants, the gift shops, and all that I know is going on above me on the pier seems to be an accepted part of this wonderful experience. I look across at the boardwalk and observe the quiet happiness that the Ferris wheel is in motion, and I feel glad that the rides are there, glad someone is riding today. Although it was never one of those things I like to do, I smile with satisfaction as I remember all the fun my children had on those rides.

As I move on to the wet sand and walk under the pier, I always have a feeling of amazement and wonder while looking down through the pilings at the ingenuity of man, who can plant high trees to such a depth so as to allow the constant pounding of the surf year after year. The smell while walking under the pier is unique; a combination of salt, sea, fish, old rotting wood, and kelp. The air under the pier is cool and damp. Reaching the other side and stepping to one side to avoid the flies hovering a deposit of seaweed kelp, I move on to the hot sand and walk toward a secluded place I have picked out all for myself. After spreading my beach towel and placing all my things on one side, I slip off my sandals and lie down on the warm sand. The sun feels especially hot on my bare back. I stir around in the sand to make a comfortable place molded to the contour of my body. Relaxation is on its way, my thoughts have a way of turning to feelings of thankfulness for such a place as the beach, and my gratitude is transformed to prayer as I visit for a while with the Lord of all this grandeur. Listening to the sound of the surf, I finally fall asleep. After a while the sound of children splashing and playing awakens me, and I know I should turn over. I raise my head to look above at the hotel and the surfers running down toward the beach with their surfboards under their arms. What a joy it is to watch strong, young, brown bodies who have the strength to challenge fearlessly the treachery of the sea.

After I have lain on my back long enough to become extremely warm, I decide it is time to cool off and take a dip. The water is cold, so I go in slowly, watching enviously as some youngsters skim across the water and dive in. There is not a feeling in all the world like the ocean as it moves away from your feet and the sand gives way beneath. I reach down to scoop a handful of wet sand as the tide goes out and show a child nearby all the little sand crabs who live so close to the surface just underfoot. Then I drop them and they disappear quickly into the wet sand as if they were only a dream.

Since it is getting late in the day and the beach is beginning to be quieter of people, I decide to dry off by walking along the beach. The water reaches up from time to time to touch my toes. Other times I run out to meet it and splash along for a while. There is a fog moving in, adding its peaceful aura to the quiet of late afternoon. A fishing boat is heading toward the pier. The sails on boats far out in the lagoon seem to become larger as they move in toward home. Looking along the cliffs, I remember the day I climbed to the top and watched heavy surf and white foam from one side and a quiet lagoon on the other. I look across the wide expanse of ocean, and wonder what my son, so many miles across the water, is doing at this moment. As I turn toward home, I watch a man with a metal detector combing the sand, and I wonder how many pop tops he picked up before he found a coin. The laughter has quieted on the boardwalk, but the Ferris wheel still turns and when I arrive at the step, tired but refreshed, I felt a wave of love of life, the world, and people sweep peacefully over me. Time seems to stand suspended, all cares of the world somehow forgotten or misplaced for another time, another place. The lights seem to have an iridescent glow.

At the conclusion of this adventure in memory, I am relaxed. You can choose any memory you have had. A trip to the beach may not mean anything to you. The more often you do this, the more you will realize just how many really good things happened in your life. You will look forward to making more good memories. This can also be done in a positive way as an adventure into the future to bring into being that which you first structure and plan in your mind. However you must plan and feel every detail and believe that it will come about.

Matthew states:

"And Jesus said into the Centurion, go thy way; and as thou hast believed, so be it unto thee."

This is the art of creative thinking, and it must be done in a relaxed way, in faith, believing.

Make Peace With Yourself

There is a vital, unseen force that regulates all systems and defenses which is sensitive to negative, nervous stimuli. It can be just as sensitive to positive stimuli when other positive rules are obeyed, such as correct dietary living habits, correct thinking patterns. If the

179

spiritual aura is strong, evil or negative stimuli seem to bounce off and positive, exulting thoughts are excepted, enhancing the spiritual beauty of such a person. People who feel their world with anger, insult, tension, jealousy, fear, disappointment, argument, too many people or too few people, bickering, violence, insecurity, dissatisfaction, or strife become sure prey for pain and sorrow. Panic and uncertainty spread gradually rejecting all possibility for a solution. The bitter contest begins between which circumstance or which person can be blamed for the now acknowledged failure. They will say "I didn't have a fair chance," "I had not skill; I wasn't clever," "I had a poor home life," "I was not understood," "I was not loved." Their grievances toward society are endless. There aura shrinks to a repellent, muddy green and never do they once consider that the fault was theirs.

To have energy of spirit we must be continually receiving and absorbing beautiful, positive, uplifting thoughts and auto suggestions both from outside and inside ourselves. The words that fall from our tongues, the reflections we radiate from our beings must be within the bounds of righteous purity and love for all living things that exist around us. Would you deliberately give an autosuggestion to someone you loved that could cause them to be ill or to die? And yet this is how people whose tongues are not guarded lay a path of devastation and waste before them.

There is also a type of person who lives a fairly good life but does not ever seek to guard the tongue. Without computed segregation, everything that comes into the head falls out of the mouth. They cause much pain to others but often think of themselves as honest.

When we learn to adjust our computer to accept or reject correctly and give out from ourselves information or autosuggestion that will bless rather than destroy, we will be on our way to peace

In order to find peace of soul, many other factors are involved. All things in our lives must be subjected to restriction where discipline must be more and more stringent. When the laws of peace are observed, the way is narrow but the opening above and beyond is wide and vast, filled with peace and happiness. Those who think peace can be secured by doing anything they please to themselves or others, only find the road to pain.

It has been wisely and anonymously said:

"He who loses the power of discrimination loses all."

Theosophic systems of philosophy or religion, which claim to have the special insight and power of the divine nature achieved through spiritual self-development, have a way of trapping those who feel hopeless as they view the world situation. Those who become deeply involved in such philosophies can by the power of darkness, perform signs that astound and convert. For the most part, metaphysicians as a class, merely waste their time building mystic, philosophic systems the way children build blocks, and they eventually lose themselves in a jungle of verbal speculation, useless to themselves and to the world except as mental exercise. They seem to destroy eventually their ability to analyze, discriminate, or discern. This, of course, is what Satan wishes to achieve in their lives. Petrify the minds of the wanderers, leave them sitting on a cushion doing their gymnastic meditations or wandering in circles hoping to gain the power.

Power is what this quest is all about, not a power over oneself which can only be achieved by living in association with people and life circumstances, but a power given of evil to those who are not stupid enough to remain on the cushion without some manifestation or some reward. Metaphysics does not destroy faith, as faith is also a requirement to receive such Satanic power. It does, however, corrupt and distort the religious spirit because it causes the men who become involved to become selfish and self-centered with a goal to be serene under all circumstances. This is what is bringing us more often to the idea, "do your own thing." What would happen to the world if everyone turned to this worship of individualism? Who would ever take care of anyone else? We see on all sides the neglected little ones and the breakdown in family life, whose parents are on a drug kick or have advanced to cushion meditation. This is a world of motion, and when we become quietly involved in self, atrophy of the spirit sets in. We no longer care about others, only self and self pleasure. The grandest nobility of man is on the move always – some of the time outside of himself and some of the time within, where both factors working together bring him to perfection.

Michelangelo said:

"Trifles make perfection and perfection is no trifle."
Thinking, weighing, analyzing, discriminating, discerning, calculating, creating, dreaming and planning are important building blocks of perfection.

Ralph Waldo Emerson said:

"I count him a great man who inhabits a higher sphere of thought, into which other men rise with difficulty and labor."

To do nothing but meditate, to bring about only psychic wonder is like the performance of a magician. Of what value to the individual has the performance been? It becomes an ego trip, it becomes a power struggle. Power to do what? Show forth to others. So what? Who needs it except perhaps to be entertained. The real need is inside. Who am I? What have I done with what I have? Whom have I served? Whom have I helped? What have I learned? The great struggle – and it is a very real struggle – is between good and evil. The common good for all. The egomaniac triviality and cleverness will not carry a man's name down through the corridors of time, permanently edging his name in the rock of ages.

Amiel said:

"Cleverness is useful in everything sufficient to nothing."

It is what he has done for the world. The man who has done the greatest good for the most people in his generation (and for generations to come) is the one most cherished and remembered. If we must have a quest, let it be the pursuit of truth. This is all that was made to endure. To seek only after power is a wasteful delusion.

Power rises and falls while truth remains. The acquisition of truth and knowledge can be a game far more fascinating and lasting than the quest for money or power. To turn that knowledge into service for each other's prosperity, peace, and help for all.

The problem we have today (as always) is caused from those who seek wealth and power, who have lost that special sensitivity to people around them as they plow through, over, and past. Those people who stomp on everything that is really love and tender happiness cast the largest shadow on world peace. Nothing says we cannot find this peace within, even though the struggle is like two dogs fighting over a bone that goes on all around us. It's a matter of harmony.

Francis bacon said:

> *"No pleasure is comparable to standing upon a vantage ground of truth – a hill not to be commanded where the air is always clear and serene – and see the error and wanderings and mist and tempest in the vale below."*

Down through history we find those few who have stood upon this vantage ground of truth. Let me quote what Carlyle said of Coleridge and his metaphysics. See if you can understand what he is saying from his vantage point.

> *"His life had been an abstract thinking and dreaming, idealistic passed amid the ghosts of defunct bodies and unknown ones. The moaning sing-song of that theosophic metaphysical monotony left on you at last a very dreary feeling – but in general, you could not call this aimless, cloud-clapped, cloud-based lawlessly meandering human discourse of reason by the name of 'excellent talk' but only 'surprising' and were reminded bitterly of Hazlitt said of it 'excellent talker very – if you let him start from no premises and come to no conclusion.'*
> *"The truth is I now see Coleridge's talk and speculation as the emblem of himself; in it as incompetent*

maniacs or of cynical charlatans deliberately bent on buncoing the public by turning rational form full of spiritual emotion into 'significant or imagined form' full of aesthetic emotion which no one comprehends except the artistic crooks who fabricate it, perhaps to swindle the cunningly bewildered portion of the world – in him a ray of heavenly inspiration struggled, in a tragically ineffectual degree, with weakness of flesh and blood he preferred to create logical Fata Morganas of himself on the hither side, and laboriously solace himself with these, and he had not valiantly grappled with it; he had fled from it: sought refuge in vague daydreams, hollow compromises in opium, in theosophic metaphysics – and so the empyrean element lying smothered under the terrene and yet inextinguishable there made sad writhings. For the old eternal powers do live forever; nor do their laws know any change; however, we in our poor wig and church trippets may attempt to read their law. To steal into heaven by the modern method, of sticking ostrich-like your head into fallacies on earth, equally as by ancient and by all conceivable methods is forever forbidden. High treason is the name of that attempt, and it continues to punish as such. Strange enough: here once more was a kind of Heaven-scaling Juno; and to him, as to the old one the just gods were very Stern! The ever-revolving, never advancing wheel (of a kind) was his through life; and from his cloud Juno did not heed to procreate strange centaurs, special Puseyism's, monstrous illusory Hybrids, and ecclesiastical chimeras which now roam the earth in a very lamentable manner?"

This was preached at Coleridge's funeral. What a sendoff and yet I see youngsters all around me today with the same misguided attitude fleeing from reality and truth into fables – allowing the drugs in the immorality of flesh to smother the light that burned once within them. What a waste!

Note:

Centaurs: Greek monsters of legend

Chimeras: horrible creatures of imagination; absurd, impossible ideas; wild fancy.

There can be no peace in the world until there is peace in all people, but there can be no peace in all the people because each is at a different stage of development and accomplishment in obedience to the laws that exist. We have been given free agency to choose, and choose we must. In so choosing, we place ourselves in chaos or harmony. The only way to internal peace is by obedience to the laws which are eternal. When we do not understand the law we are still buffeted by that law, even though at times we may obey. We still suffer as we swing back and forth from obedience to disobedience in a game of chance.

Until we pay close attention to trial and error we cannot find the secret law requires. Even in searching we are buffeted about. Therefore, there can be no peace until we learn the law and obey it. When it takes a lifetime to learn, there can be no real joy in only those moments here and there when we were in harmony.

It is like learning to walk: the baby who learns fastest and best avoids the most bumps. If we want to have less bumps, we will learn the fastest and best way to obey that which we learn to be true. When we learn a truth and refuse to obey it we not only suffer physically but spiritually as well.

Russell Cornwell said:

"You may talk of Gettysburg's, 'Bloody angle' or Waterloo's 'Sunken Road' but in man's life there is no battle more severe, and no victory more Honorable than when a man fights with himself and wins the victory. Victory over oneself is the greatest feat in the world and surely he who cannot control himself, cannot control other people."

J. M. Gibby said in his book *Sand for the Rails:*

"You may escape the immediate punishment for your transgressions of law but you cannot elude the immutable sting of its gathered power."

A man does not suddenly become a thief, an adulterer, a murderer, a homosexual. Past thoughts and actions have brought him to that place where he stands today.

Gibby says:

"Natural death is a gradual process; only its consummation seems sudden."

The evil or the good man is in a gradual process as a result of choosing. If peace is what you desire, make peace first with yourself. To make peace with oneself and live on a higher vantage point we must first learn what the law requires of us and then obey it. Only then will we place ourselves in harmony where peace, perfection, and happiness dwell. We can become resigned to our fate and say we are at peace, but this is not true peace. True peace overcomes all obstacles and is not resignation. True peace is only won on the battlefield of the soul: respecting justice and obeying the law. Having hope of mercy and the courage to go on, thus exhibiting faith in a righteous God who has a correct reason for all of this.

In John 16:33, Christ said:

"These things I have spoken unto you, that ye might have peace. In the world ye shall have tribulations: but be of good cheer; I have overcome the world."

The world is full of sick people, sick not only in body but in spirit. They devote their entire lives to seeking after lies instead of truth, who delight in inflicting injury, physically or prejudiciously upon others. They surround themselves with wild abuse. They fill their hearts with blaming others, quarreling, cursing, nagging, and fighting. They criticize and pick at others. With this kind of an aura surrounding their lives, they are quickly attracted to the other negative forces about them, responding to them. Their world begins to be filled with greed, falsehood, hypocrisy, perjury, miserliness, robbery, bribery, trickery, and meanness. The world is filled to overflowing with this kind of sickness and when the world at different periods in history has become ripened in iniquity, a purging takes place and the wicked again blame God for all their problems. This may be compared to a cold when the waste and the filth reaches such a stage as to destroy all life on earth an elimination is forced to rid the earth of corruption that some may remain and live. To me it is as simple as that, and man, by his wrong choices, as in diet, has brought himself to such a point as to be under such condemnation.

Men who wish to live right, somehow become a party to the wickedness of those in power over them medically, as we have seen in our generation. We all seem to be tainted and entangled in the net of the power mongers and their intrigues, and we know not that Satan controls the money of the world and uses us like pawns in a game to further his plan of hate and contempt upon us.

The only way out is through the prayer of faith, courage, a cheerful countenance, and obedience to that which is good. These things will raise us above the storm into a place of peace and happiness.

In Doctrine & Covenants 90:24 it says:

> *"Search diligently, pray always, and be believing, and all things shall work together for your good, if ye walk uprightly and remember the covenant wherewith ye have covenanted one with another."*

When we develop a strong and beautiful aura, the negative things of the world cannot penetrate to hurt us. Observe, as you mingle among people and listen to the average conversation which dwells upon negative evils, just how few there are who stand out in a positive, beautiful way. These few seem to reflect a contagious enthusiasm. The personality is magnetic and hypnotic. Their conversation is joyous and stimulating, happy in all respects. They are mentally alert to everyone. When they walk into a group of people, the whole room seems to come alive with the glow of their presence. They are a joy to everyone. They are the oasis in the desert. Everyone is drawn like a magnet to such a person the same way we are repelled by the sick and negative person. In order to be well we must emulate them. We must learn to be of good cheer.

In John 14:27 Christ said:

"... Let not your heart be troubled, neither let it be afraid."

Worry and fear are bitter enemies to good health. The world is aglow with love, beauty, happiness. It's a matter of seeking it out, expecting it and enjoying it. Fear destroys health. Faith builds health.

When we seek to find health and learn about nature's medicines, it is because we are more positive than most and are being led along to a solution. As we learn to obey the rules, we find truth upon truth, knowledge upon knowledge until we come to perfect knowledge.

On the other hand, those who are negative follow all the wrong paths to health, paying the high medical costs, suffering great pain, and these because they refused to discover the laws of health. Judgment extracts its final penalty – usually with great anguish.

Often sadness is caused by those whom we love most who may be deeply entangled in evil. Our hearts are torn because of them but the scriptures tell us, in Psalm 55:22:

"Cast thy burden upon the Lord, and he shall sustain thee: he shall never suffer the righteous to be moved."

We do not always take this literally and turn those we love, who cause us pain, to the Lord to let him deal with them. Often, if we have to watch, we cannot stand the chastisement they must go through, and we continually beg for mercy, thus extending the time of our worry. We actually reject all possibility for solution, whereas if we allowed to happen what could be done in their behalf it may be solved sooner than we could solve it. It's like a mother hovering over a spoiled child with permissive indulgence, refusing to allow the father to punish him. Prayers of the faithful are heard, respected, and answered. We must take care, therefore, in what we ask regarding the wayward members of our families, who tear at our heartstrings.

If it were possible – and it can be if we try – we must learn to turn off those things we cannot solve and pass them on to a higher intelligence than our own – solve the things we can, and cheerfully and patiently wait.

Patients, this is a problem. To wait on the Lord in faith, knowing all things are done for our good, growth, and development, is the easiest way to wait. This is a part of the test of a cheerful person. A woman I know who has been through more than most people have ever gone through because of her loved ones, still maintains her sense of humor. She always leaves me with a grateful feeling for the strength and faith she exhibits. Happy are people like her who set such examples of faith and good cheer.

We must continually try to be cheerful, even if at first it seems foreign to our nature, put on, or affected. This is how faith and all other positive attributes we may admire in others are built. Often the negative person will say about a cheerful person, "she has all the luck," or "he had everything to begin with." Not so; these attributes are earned and worked for in this world or the world before, they are not given by chance.

Brigham Young, *Journal of Discourses 9:244,* said:

"When man is industrious and righteous, then is he happy."

He also said in *Journal of Discourses 6:41:*

"You never saw a true Saint in the world that had sorrow, neither can you find one. If persons are destitute of the fountain of living water, or the principles of eternal life, then they are sorrowful. If the words of life dwell with us,

and we have hope of eternal life and glory, and let that spark within us kindle a flame, to the consuming of the least and last remains of selfishness, we never can walk in darkness and are strangers to doubt and fear."

Sometimes we feel very close to the Lord and at other times we feel far from him. The Lord does not move; it is we who rise and fall.

If you are going to fly a small plane, you would first call the tower and they would give you the direction and speed of the winds aloft. You have a slide computer and you would compute your compass angle. In order to arrive at a certain point by travel, the winds aloft will try to carry you in their direction, drifting you off course, so you must fly into the wind or what is described as "crabbing into the wind." How much you must crab into the wind is determined by how hard the wind is pushing you off course and the angle of direction. As you cross each checkpoint in your flight plan or each city you observe below, you can determine if you have computed correctly. If the winds have blown you off course you will then make the correction. If you have certain omnidirectional radio equipment aboard your plane, you can determine where you are without visual reference.

In this life we live with a constant opposition like the winds aloft which can push us off our course.

The Scriptures, the great literature, the books and knowledge of past trial and error are the laws we draw from to compute our course. Then if we have omnidirectional equipment or the ability to tap into infinite intelligence through faith, we can determine where we are at all times without visual reference.

Life is a constant struggle to correct. Into error, back to correct course, and so on from birth to death. How well we maintain a correct course determines how happy, healthy and successful we are. Herbs have a way of correcting all systems, a way of placing the body back on a correct course.

The answer to health does not lie completely, however, in the taking of medicines, even though a generous God has allowed us a way out with herbs when we obey, the same as he allows us to faint when we have endured the highest pitch of pain to our individual limit. God has given us varying degrees of pain, but never causes us to suffer any higher than a certain level and leaves it to us how long we are willing to suffer that high pitch of pain before we faint.

We are, however, expected to live the law. We are expected to find out what that law is. Often we seek in all the wrong directions and observe not nature in all its beauty as it moves and has its being in everything that surrounds us.

The laws of Revelation are exact and based upon faith. When we develop sufficient faith, answers will come and we will hear, rejoice, and by obedience we will correct the error and find ourselves back on course.

Hippocrates said:

"Use gentle treatment and try to encourage the natural healing process.
"Plants also have mystical properties in a most wonderful degree – herbs are secrets of dreams and enchantments."

Thomas Edison said:

"The Doctor of the future will give no medicine but will interest his patients in the care of the human frame and in the cause of prevention of disease."

CHAPTER 5

OLD BOOKS

Adolf Hitler said:

"If you tell a lie big enough, and long enough, and often enough, the people will believe it."

Reading the old medical books has proven to me, we have been told too many lies for too long, and we need to take a new look at what some of the past physicians had to say. This chapter will give some writings from old books.

It may interest you to know what some of the authors of the old books wrote, aside from those listed in the section on herbs.

Doctor William Salmon, 1675-1708 (Polygraphic), was probably one of the most interesting scholars I studied in the old books because his knowledge is so widespread: drawing, painting, making and mixing paint as well as liquid gold and silver for paint, the coloring and dying of metal, cloth, silk, bone, wood and glass, and making and using varnish, perfume, powders, soaps, balsam inks, sealing wax, and artificial pearls. He even wrote on palmistry. His other books on herbal medicine, complete with case histories, and medical books for physicians, prove to me his ability as a physician.

Some case histories in his *Paralaremata* show that he often used a laxative first, then a specific herbal formula. The results are very interesting and prove to me again that what I say in my book *Is Any Sick Among You?* is true.

Dr. Salmon's *Family Dictionary* gives recipes for cakes, pies, puddings, methods to prepare meat, how to make pickles, etc.

In his book *Old Medical Instruments,* he talks about coughs, difficult breathing (pages 15-93) and catarrh, relating how to make a cough drop with horehound, sugar, licorice, and oil of cinnamon.

He uses the word "laudanum" for opiate, an old-fashioned word not much in use today. In his book *Practice of Physick* (1979, page 75), speaking of the disease of pleurisy, he makes an interesting comment, that if pleurisy exceeds the 14th day, it evolves into emphysema, consumption or putrid ulcers.

Sometimes I feel we do not pay enough attention to the discomfort of acute pleurisy occurring along with a cold condition. In using the drugs that force chronic waste back into the body when it is attempting to eliminate, we do exactly what he suggests, creating in ourselves those chronic diseases he mentions.

When writing in his book *Practice of Physick* (pages 64, 66, 67) his observation on rheumatism is that after fever is gone, pain is translated to some new place in the body. Blood-letting, he says, is sometimes fatal to this disease especially. Also, the very young, old, fat or consumptive are susceptible, so he suggests lemon, water Lilies, Violet, purges, laxatives, Saffron, or Rosemary rather than blood-letting. On page 592 in his writing on ulcers he follows a similar method as do physicians today by avoiding fruits and vegetables and using meats, eggs, grain, gruel and broths. Since this method would not be so seemingly irritating to the stomach, this has been the obviously logical method to follow. When we understand fully how the body feeds and eliminates, we know that this method only prolongs the disease.

Joseph Smith in *The Dogmaticus or Family Physician* (1829) in his Preface said:

"Ever since the first introduction of moral evil into the world, man has been a subject of misery and disease: or sickness, pain and death, are the very fruits of sin. All have sinned, and have come short of the glory of God! So much that every subject of sin is, more or less, a subject of disease.

"And when we take a view of the human machine, and it's curious mechanism, we are at once struck with wonder and surprise, and must say with the psalmist, "how wondrous are thy works, oh Lord. How strange that a harp of a thousand strings, should keep in tune so long." But we are workmanship of God's hand, and well calculated to live long upon the earth and every nerve and every string would keep their regular motion, and the blood would run its rounds until the appointed time, were it not for some obviating or irritating power, that may consist in, or proceed from, contagion, poison, contusion, pressure, or retention of some natural evacuations, etc.

"Life and death, then are on condition of man's obedience or disobedience, and he that would live long on the earth, and enjoy good health, must observe the rules of morality and true piety – be temperate in all things, from his youth to his grave.

"But as this is not generally the case, it is become a subject of great importance to each individual, to know how he may alleviate those distressing pains, that so torment and rack his mortal frame. God has not left us in a situation in which we are subject to so many diseases without providing a remedy.

"But ignorance and superstition prevails so abundantly among the people, that many of them not only suffer on a long and tedious bed of sickness, but have to

expend the last cent they possess, to satisfy their attending physician.

"Let wisdom speak, and she will say, that medicine, like religion, is free for every man. The insignificant animals, even the toads, if bitten by any poisonous animal, fly to the antidote which, to them proves a sure remedy."

On page 15: Glands – When obstructed become large and endurates; from which scherrus and cancers are produced.

On page 32: he understood very well that when any organ of elimination was obstructed, that disease was the result. He understood that to overcome the disease, the obstruction must be removed, the bowel, kidney and skin opened to eliminate.

On pages 39-40: he lists treatment for contagious disease and refers to the use of Lobelia as emetick laxatives and saffron.

On pages 41-42: for chronic disease he recommends mandrake, goldenseal and blood root and if the pulse is weak, cayenne. He recommends diuretics and poultices.

On page 44: for eruptions he recommends again saffron, sarsaparilla, laxatives, ointments, and salves.

For external inflammation: poultices, plasters, water therapy, and again that the bowel be kept open.

He says on page 49 that for inflammatory disease, "open pores at the surface, cleanse stomach and bowels, and produce and maintain a general action through the system."

On page 51, for spasmodick disease, such as asthma, croup, convulsions, spasms, lockjaw, etc., he recommends the antispasmodic tincture.

Page 118: at the commencement of disease by cleansing the stomach and bowels by taking suitable emeticks and catharticks, or both if necessary, and opening the pores of the surface, either by taking sweating medicines, or steaming over hot Hemlock tea or both, if needful, we stop the progress of disease in time, preserve health, and save much pain and expense.

The Dr. Joseph Smith is not the Mormon prophet, even though his book was printed in Rochester, New York. The Prophet, however was well acquainted with the use of herbs. His father was involved in a Mercantile career which invested heavily in shipments of Ginseng root to China. In the *History of the LDS church,* volume 5, page 126, I quote:

In his diary the Prophet notes that:

"He was suddenly and severely attacked by disease, with strong symptoms of apoplexy."

And then adds:

"We immediately administered to him by the laying on of hands and prayer accompanied with herbs."

He also mentions the use of Lobelia on page 232 under date 26 December 1842:

"General law gave me in custody of Doctor Richards, with whom I visited sister Morey, who was severely afflicted. We prescribed Lobelia for her among other things which is excellent in its place."

He said in the *Documentary history of the LDS Church* also, 4:414:

"I preached to a large congregation at the stand on the science and practice of medicine, desiring to persuade the Saints to trust in God when sick, and not in the arm of flesh. And led by faith, and not by medicine or poison: When they were sick and had called for the elders to pray for them, and they were not healed to use herbs and mild food."

196

Benjamin Smith Barton in *Collection for and Essay Materia Medica* (1798) said in Part II, page XI:

"No candid physician will deny that he often meets with cases in which the choice of active medicines is a matter of consequences. So various are the forms under which diseases present themselves, that it becomes absolutely necessary to know, and to possess, a great number of different medicines, even of those which are endowed with a common assemblage of properties."

He said of "Geranium":

"This is, certainly a vegetable entitled to the attention of American Physicians, a powerful astringent for Venereal disease."

In referring to the Indians and their medicines, many of the herbs he writes about our names unknown to me.

If the botanist would only begin to seek out the medical history of all early American and Indian history and begin a systematic testing of the herbals, many wonderful things would be revealed.

So many of the botanical names have been changed with time and translation from one language to another it is hard to identify many names used in the old books. However, some have always remained the same and have been shown to be used for the same purpose in the art of healing, year after year, until our own time.

James C. Jackson, in *How Treat the Sick Without Medicine* (1870), said:

"Gluttony is a very great cause of disease. It is a prevalent vice with our people."

On page 235 he said:

"Tea, coffee, tobacco, pepper, mustard, salt, flesh meat, will create such a condition of the organic nerves, and the mucous lining of his stomach, as to re-establish the desire for liquor, and then we will drink come what may to his pledges or social position."

Phelps Brown, in *Complete Herbalist, People Their Old Physicians* (1881), said:

"The Lord has created medicine out of the earth, and he that is wise will not abhor them."

On page 11 he maintained that the surest and safest way to overcome disease was with herbal medicine, not chemical science.

"I stoutly contend that all such organic substances are taken up by plants and distributed the various tissues and elements of the human being, either in the way of food or medicine, in exactly the precise quantity requisite for man's perfect health, if rightly used."

He said they are prepared and eliminated in a way far superior to anything conceived by man and chemical science.

John Pechey (1655-1716) in *The Storehouse of Physical Practice* gave a purge to clear the body in the case of eye problems – This is made into a syrup with liquor and syrup of roses:
> Senna
> Fennel
> Betony
> Eyebright
> Vervain

On page 76 for hearing, deafness – to this add wine and poor warm into the ear:
> Marjoram
> Wormwood
> Pennyroyal
> Thyme

Sage
Mint
Marshmallow
Chamomile
Rosemary
Cinnamon
Clove

On page 91 for ulcers of the nostrils:
Pomegranate peel
Plantain
Horsetail
Mouse-ear
Rupture wart

It is interesting that most of the old books agree that purging in cases of gonorrhea or syphilis causes it to become worse. It is my opinion, as I have said before in my book *Is Any Sick Among you?*, that venereal disease is a disease of malnutrition as well as sin. When the body is purged, even more body nutrients are lost causing weakness.

John Newton (1622-1678), wrote *Cosmographia*. He wrote on geometry, geography, astronomy, and calendars.

William Cockburn (1669-1739), in *Symptoms of Nature Causes and Cure of Gonorrhea*, talks about a green liquid on page 43:

"Tis well-known that true pus of gonorrhoea is only generated in muscles and muscular parts, and the further any part recedes from being muscular, the less apt is pus to be generated in that part"

On page 122 he talked about a formula. Purging medicines do not cure; they only weaken fibers and cause running in greater quantity.

Harvey Gideon (1640-1700) wrote *The Conclave of Physicians* into parts. On page 3 he quoted Ecclesiastes 2:3 where it mentions a time to kill and a time to heal:

> *"It highly concerns the duty of every honest and conscientious Physician, to contribute to his Faculty, what may tend to the promoting and advancement of it; which, in my judgment, can best be performed by making practical observations, to the end the time of killing may be avoided. Furthermore observe that as Solomon sits down, that there is a time to kill, before time to heal: so generally Physicians (especially of pretended societies) kill more than they cure."*

He stated on page 5 that in most countries a criminal who is to be put to the rack, or anyways executed, is usually, from his suffering called the patient or sufferer; and so the sick man that is to subject himself to the rigid sentence of the combined Physicians, which renders the word Patient or Suffer truly synonymous for both.

On pages 6 and 7 he compared a group of Physicians to a jury, who without examination convict a person of disease, tell them that they are going to die, then by bleeding too much, execute the person.

On page 10 he said that it was named by his men of Physick, the new disease: a name of ignorance, on their accustomed *Asylum ignorantie,* to which they take their refuge, when they know not what the disease is, or what to call it. One time they shall tell you it is an Ague; another it is a fever; a third, it's an Ague and fever; a fourth, it's fever and Ague; a fifth, it's the new disease.

On page 11 he talks about Physicians who make a mistake and somebody suffers. The story is quieted so the Physician does not lose his status, and law shelters him from scandal.

He said on page 49 that some physicasters, by reputing themselves virtuosos, mathematicians, philosophers, and witty cracks, have insinuated this Enthymeme to the commonality, that therefore they must necessarily arrive to the top of their profession; for since there porous brain was capable of imbibing some knotty mysteries, it's not improbable they might much earlier suck up the quintessence of the art of medicine.

Thomas Coche (1675) wrote for the poor of the town and country. On page 25 he said:

"Those who have imperfect health, or are under any manifest disease, and eat much and get little strength by eating, tis a sign they have themselves to too full a diet: and the more you cram and cherish such bodies, the less they shall thrive by it but grow worse and worse, because, by much feeding, you do but increase the vitiated and bred humours, which should be wasted by bleeding, purging or abstinence."

He writes on page 26 against nurses, etc., trying to feed the sick, first one good thing and then another.

On page 28 he said:

"If you eat a large breakfast eat no dinner: if you eat no dinner eat an early supper: if you eat an early supper eat no breakfast: if no breakfast eat an early dinner and by this means you will keep your stomach clean, strong and vigorous and preserve thereby a good digestion, distribution of your food."

He said on page 29:

"Keep constantly to a plain, simple and single diet: none enjoy more health, and live longer, than those that avoid variety and curiosity of meats and drinks which only serve to entice us to our own ruine."

On page 42 he also talks about the steam baths to throw off poisons and venom from the blood.

Colon

William Cockburn (1669-1739) in *Account of Nature, Symptoms and Cure,* mentions that Vander Heyden, the city physician of Ghent, was the first to bring Whey or Whey clysters into vogue. We still use Whey for help with colon and related problems. Today we use acidophilus culture, Whey, yogurt, or B_6 when the colon has been ulcerated or filled with cancer and no longer produces its own B_6.

When the body is unable to produce B_6, digestion is impaired and other nutrients are not properly used.

Fever

Henry Burdon (1743) in *The Fountain of Health,* writes on fire, pleurisy, measles, doubt and dropsy. He said that saffron, peony waters, and black cherry would correct acidity in the stomach. He speaks of senna and rhubarb to open the body and states on page 6 that sickness is caused from being overfed. Along with all others who wrote on medicine, he did not want to be accused of quackery. He seemed to worry about danger to himself without someone to sponsor him. In that time a Doctor would usually write a book for some prominent person, thus receiving approval of the populace.

That sicknesses is caused from being overfed, we can readily see in our day, with so much food available.

He calls the dread of death a malignant fever and brings on death by fear. His idea about malignant fever has been well proven among those who deal with the sickness of the mind. We can think ourselves into and out of many things. Health is so often relative to our attitude of mind.

William Cockburn (1669-1739) in *Account of Nature, Symptoms and cure,* on pages 32 and 33, he shows how purging relieves fevers and emetic medicines relieve seasickness. He noted they were all right after cleansing unless they again ate salt and beef or meat. Then sickness would begin again.

He observed in his Preface, Verse VIII:

"This increase of disease and medicines has another effect. For diseases did not become numerous, but mixed also with one another, that it was not easy to distinguish them.

"Now whether these strange and different successes were owing to any mistake in judging the distemper and miss application of medicines or that the nature of the disease did not continue to be the same, gave occasion to new inquiries and much speculation"

On pages 241 and 242 he stated that he gave vomits and purges for dysentery with success.

On page 31 he said that:

"Hippocrates observes that a loathing of food is an ill sign when anyone has been long ill of dysentery, but a worse sign if attended with fever."

On page 6 he stated:

"Tis true, salt rituals have been found, by experience, the worst of all others to digest.

He stated on pages 26 and 27 how easily the people catch cold:

"Yet I cannot forbear observing, that an untimely use of sweating medicines in some thickening lozenges in others is more frequently the productive cause of fevers phthysicks and of more fatal consequence than a cold could have been if left to the strength of the blood and abstinence, without employing any other auxiliaries."

On page 97 he talks about fevers being cured by putting the patient in water:

"Where sailors have fallen overboard in the delirious fever and are afterward taken out they begin to sweat."

He describes on page 100 how purging relieves fever.

On page 122 he stated that powders were used instead of teas placed in water.

William Salmon in *Synopsis Medicinae* (1681): he mentions attacking of doctors in his preface and uses the original manuscript of Paracelus. He also talks of the problems of being a doctor and his conflicts.

Page 43, preface:

"There is scarcely indeed any worthy thing that can escape the lash of these profane and licentious tongues... For they speak well of nothing but what is likely to agree with their pernicious appetites."

He was concerned about any errors but asks the reader to accept any errors as unintentional. He invites lovers of learning to correct the author as he will be glad to find it out.

His observations were:

Chapter XXXVII, verse XVII:

"Obstruction is the stoppage of the inwards by thickened phlegm so that they cannot execute their office."

Chapter XXXVII, verse XIX:

"When the gall is obstructed it causeth the Yellow Jaundice, when the spleen – the Black Jaundice.

Chapter XXXVII, verse XX:

"Lastly, when the pipes of the urine or bladder are stopped it is by reason of gravel or the stone, which

obstruction, by reason of their sharpness, cause extreme pain."

Page 163 he mentions a hardening of the liver or spleen or both (cachexia) "bad digestion, loathing of meat and desire of drink." He said:

"Old men and children are chiefly afflicted herewith. Watery humor through the whole body for want of nourishment."

This is an interesting observation – without a knowledge of vitamin values and very correct.

William Salmon in *Systema Medicinale* (1686):

"Tincture of Benzoin: Much to be said for their heating and cooling the body in disease. Certain herbs have these abilities."

Herman Boerhaave (1668-1738), *Institutions in Physick*, collected from writings of the most eminent physicians.

On page 289 he suggested a diet for health:
    Lean meat
    Vegetables – breadroots and fruit
    Simple food dry and hard and difficult to putrefaction
    Milk in childhood and sparing cold water

His suggestions are very good for a normal diet. In correct combinations they would be right. Then of course, chronic illness would require the mild foods and herbs.

Edmund Borlase (1882) in *Latham Spaw* on page 17 states that drinking mineral water from a spaw acts as a diuretic. Within an hour and a half, 2 chambers were filled with urine.

On page 25 he says that instead of the water, fennel seeds, coriander seeds, lemon or orange peel, Angelica root, or roots of candied Enula Campana can be taken with the mineral water, which brings off the water gradually.

On page 27:

"In a weaker body, Manna may be sufficient, rhubarb, with Cream of Tartar, or my De-obstructive powder which I have observed hath done singularly well."

On page 31 he recommends mild exercise with the drinking of the water. If a person sweats, some of the water is lost, so riding, shooting, or bowling is recommended, just enough to get the circulation going, and distribute the water throughout the body.

He talks about colic and itch on page 46.

He says on page 52 that a man had a lot of pain in his legs and feet. He crawled to the spaw and drank some of the water, then took some home with him. The next morning, his legs were broken out with a lot of pimples, which expelled much water.

On page 60 he talks about ulcers.

He writes about many uses for the waters from the Spaw: sores, aches, itch, heart pains, the passage of stones, and he even says it cures aging which amused me as that would really be something to cure.

Benjamin Allen (1699), in *The Natural History of the Chalybeat and Purgin Waters of England,* talks about Scarburgh Springs in his preface. It was useful for the following problems: vertigo, cramp, colicks, jaundice, stomach, bowels, glands and kidneys, gout, diabetes, diseases proceeded by grief of mind, nervousness, stones, gas, rheumatism, inflammations, and running pains.

It has been well-known through all generations of time that water has great healing benefits. Some water has a laxative effect, and more than not, a purges is all that is needed to restore health. In grandmother's day, the first thing she would do in fever or sickness was to give a laxative and an enema.

John Jacob Berlu's *Treasury of Drugs Unlocked* (1733) is a full and true description of all sorts of drugs and chemical preparations, sold by druggists. It tells how to know the place of their growth, whence they came, and how to distinguish the good from the bad.

> *"Very useful for All Gentlemen, Merchants, Druggists, Doctors, Apothecaries, Chiurgeons, and there Apprentices. As also for all Travelers, Seaman, Custom house Officers, and all others that either Traffick in them, or make any Use of them, or those that import or deliver any of them at the Water-side. With a compleat Catalog of all Drugs, & c."*

Herbs were called drugs in that time, and so we now have the confusion today between the chemical or the herbal drug.

Joannes Groenevelt (b. 1647) in *Lithologia* on page 53 states:

> *"That Spirit of Nilrum does break a stone of man's body when it is out of the body is most certain and experienced. But such a quantity thereof as is requisite hereunto, is not at all to be given or injected into the human body."*

On page 59 he said:

> *"But when the stone in the bladder is greater than can by any art be forced away, there being no medicine in nature of virtue to dissolve it, the extremity of the disease requires the last and most dangerous remedy which is Exsection."*

Today doctors know not much more than Joannes Groenevelt. A kidney stone is an easy thing to dissolve with lemon juice.

Joannes Groenevelt in *Lithologia*, on page 23, says that much of the cause of stones is the constant use of beef, pork, and goat flesh and meats, salted and smoked, ducks, geese, waterfowl, unripe fruits, new beer, tartarus wines, and cold water after sweating.

On page 32 he describes pathological signs of kidney stones. Use diuretic herbs and anodyne's to prevent pain.

Sir Kenelm Digby, in *A Discourse Concerning the Vegetation of Plants,* states on page 15:

"He will find that there is no disease in man's body, but springeth from fermentation; which when it groweth so violent and unruly, that the fermented humours can no longer be contained within their oppressed vessels, or that it is continued so long that the spirits fly quite away, and thereby deliver over the remaining mass to putrefaction and rottenness MI: death, which is an essential dissolution of the whole compound, must necessarily follow."

William Cockburn (1669), in the Preface, discusses the difference between looseness of dysentery caused by diet and that caused from a pathological cause.

On pages 64-67 he states that he understood that a physick or laxative was important in some cases to rid the body of poison, but in others too much laxative was a cause for fluid buildup in the abdominal cavity. The cause of death was due to the lack of body tone where the heart's ability to pump under such an edemic condition was retarded. He understood that the slime waste of bad humors had to be removed from the body, but if the laxative were continued too long the body's ability to recover would be limited by weakness.

This is a correct assumption and is the reason why a laxative Herb is necessary to remove cancer from the body and is best taken in a formula which has other properties that build and cleanse at the same time along with herbs that kill the cancer. This is also the reason a person who is continually on a cleanse needs additional vitamins during the process.

John Pechey (1655-1716), in *The Stone-house of Physical Practice*, on page 3 discusses madness, bleeding, vomiting, strong purges. His writings were so amusing I thought you would enjoy reading what he said.

On page 7 he discusses fits, purging, vomiting. Formula for a purge:

"Take of the Fires of Black Hellebore infused in vinegar, dried and powdered, half a dram, of Ginger half a scruple, of Salt of wormwood twelve grains, of all of Amber two drops; make a powder, give it in the pulp of a roasted Apple in the morning."

On page 8 he says:

"Take of Mans skull prepared 1 ounce, of mistletoe of the oak factitious Cinnabar, and of Elk's Hoof, each half an ounce. Dose, half a scruple or one scruple. Some find benefit by shaving the head, and by applying to the forepart of a plaster."

On page 10 he mentions convulsions in children. If there were any possibilities of a child inheriting a tendency toward convulsions, they were given a remedy shortly after birth. Then in 3 to 4 days, the roots and seeds of a male peony, along with a little Elk's hoof, were sewn in a rag, and hung around the baby's neck. The nurse was also given a formula consisting of flowers of betony, peony, rosemary, red coral, angelica, and nutmeg.

On page 13 he discusses nightmares, bleeding, some things for the head, such as amber, coral and peony. He said:

"But an orderly diet is first to be prescribed, windy meats, and such as are hard of digestion are to be avoided, and sleep must not be indulged after eating or study, and large and late suppers, and lying on the back must be forbid."

About apoplexy on page 15 he said that when a physician is first called to a patient that is seized with a sleepy disease, he must endeavor to arouse him by offering violence to all his senses; and therefore he must expose his eyes to sunbeams, or to clean light. His ears must be filled with violent noises and clamours and the sick must be sure to be called aloud by his own name. Sharp things are to be blown up his nostrils, the sense of touching is to be revived by frictious villocations, plucking of the hair, ligatures, squeezing of the fingers together, and the like.

On page 28 about catarrh he says:

"Whatever precipitates the Serum through the veins, or carries it off by stool, or by sweat is good in this case, or whatever else lessens the serum."

He says about blindness on page 32 that an obstruction is usually the cause and is accompanied by compression of the optic nerve. There is phlegm or some other matter heaped up around the optic nerve, and tumors are formed. Inflammation of the brain can also cause blindness.

On page 33 he cites an example of a man who lost his sight by a violent vomit, then regained it again by another. His explanation was this: the first vomit stirred up too much and caused an obstruction, the second evacuated the obstruction and sight was regained.

It is interesting how many of the doctors wrote about Peony for brain problems.

Daniel LeClerc (1652-1728), *The Compleat Surgeon* (3rd edition). Surgical was spelled chirurgical and yet surgery was spelled as we would spell it. He made the following statements in his book:

"Why ought a surgeon to be skillful? Because without a discerning faculty he can have no certainty in what he doth.
"Why must he be experienced? Because knowledge alone does not endure him with dexterity of hand requisite

in such a person, which cannot be acquired but by experience and manual operations."

He gives a formula as an astringent to bind wounds:

"To this purpose you may also make use of cobwebs, mill-dust, and the powder of worms, eaten oak; or else take oven soot, mix with the juice of dung of an ass or ox, adding only there to the white of an egg." (Page 182)

"Besides these remedies there are also actual and potential cauteries or simple ligatures which are infallible."

On page 183 he goes on to say that cautery is not always with fire and gives a formula using vitriol which he says may cause convulsions.

On page 183, for mortification he uses wine, wormwood, St. John's wort, rosemary, aloes, myrrh, and camphor, and saffron.

On page 185 he says that for dissolving, corroborating and allaying pain or inflammation he uses comfrey, fenugreek, saffron, oil of Bay, turpentine, wax and linseed oil. He adds to this a half pound of white lead or crude opium. He says this is frequently applied with success. What the white lead is, I do not know.

On page 186 he says to use a poultice in great wounds:
          Flower of chamomile
          Melilot
          Wormwood
          Mallow
          Marshmallow
          Seeds of cumin
          Linseed powder
          Mixed with barley meal and wine

Then he says where there is fear of gangrene add saffron, myrrh, and aloes.

On page 187 he gives a formula for cleaning the wounds, listing many herbs we would use today, such as wormwood, bugle, sanicle and horehound. However, he adds a concoction of powdered crabs' eyes be taken inwardly.

James Harvey (1700), in *Praesagium Medicum,* states on page 101:

"Everyone knows the fatality of a long continued dysentery, concerning which it may be further observed with a late author that if one in this distemper is seized with an inflammation of the tongue and difficulty swallowing there is no hope left."

It seems to have been long recognized by everyone that continual dysentery was a serious problem, and we recognize this in animals as well as people. It becomes a problem of vitality as the body is dehydrated and the minerals and vitamins are leached out of the body. Nowadays we know how to give intravenous feedings to sustain body energy, but how much better it would be to overcome the cause.

George Hartman in, *The Family Physitian* gave formula for vertigo:

      Rhubarb
      Agarich (not known)
      Senna
      Fennel
      Caraway Seed
      Ginger
      Camels hay (not known)
      Betony
      Palm
For eyewash:
      Ground Ivy
      Celandine
      Daisies
      Sugar candy
      Add pint of rose water
For ulcers of mouth and throat:

Elder flowers
Plantain
White thorn flowers
Venice soap
Mulberry syrup

BIOGRAPHICAL SKETCHES

David Abercrombie (1701)

He was a Scottish physician whose books gave him a place of honor in Haller's Bibliotheca Medicinae Practicae and some of his books were translated into French, Dutch, and German. He was a fellow of the college of physicians in Amsterdam.

In his work "Protestancy proved safer than Popery," there are some interesting things to be learned about his life.

He entered the Jesuits in France and lived among them 18 years and more "being privileged after a solemn examen capable to teach divinity and philosophy in the most renowned universities in Europe." He taught grammar in Lorraine, France, mathematics and philosophy and being graduated in physick, "I practiced it not unhappily and intend to practice it hereafter, with certain hopes, God willing, of the same success." (Pages 2-5)

William Beckett (1684-1738)

Beckett was born in Abingdon, Berkshire, England. He was well known in London as a surgeon and an enthusiastic antiquary. He was elected a fellow of the Royal society December 11, 1718.

Beckett was a surgeon for some years at St. Thomas hospital, Southwhich. He wrote 5 books, among them *New Discoveries Relating to the Cure of Cancers.*

William Cowper (1666-1709)

He was apprenticed to William Bignall, a London surgeon. He was admitted as a Barber-surgeon on March 9, 1691, and began practice in London.

Cowper wrote on anatomy and straightened out some former ideas on muscle structure. He started hard breathing in 1708, so he retired and died March 8, 1709.

William Cockburn (1669-1739)

He was the grandson of Sir William Cockburn, baronet of Ryslaw and Cockburn. His name is in the register of the University of Leyden as a student of medicine, dated May 29, 1691, at 23 years of age. It was thought that he received his M.D. but the date is not known.

Cockburn had 2 years experience as ship's doctor. He discovered a remedy for dysentery, which made him a fortune. Lord Berkeley of Stratton said that they needed a cure for dysentery, and so Cockburn's method was tried on 70 patients with remarkable success. He supplied the fleet with the medicine from then on for 40 years. He wrote books on V.D. He was married twice, first in 1689 to Mary de Baudisson, who died July 5, 1728, at age 64; then on April 5, 1729, to Lady Mary Fielding, who was a patient of his.

Cockburn is described as an old, very rich quack, and the lady was very ugly. He died at age 70, and he was buried in the middle aisle of Westminster Abbey.

Nicholas Culpepper (1616-1654)

He was born in London. He translated the *College of Physicians' Pharmacopeia* into English under the title of *A Physical Directory*. This translation was unauthorized and caused a lot of excitement at the College of Physicians, who described it as done very filthily into English, by one Nicholas Culpepper.

Such hard work and strain ruined his health, and he died of consumption at age 38. He was married and the father of 7 children. His widow said, "He left 79 books of his own making in my hands."

Nicholas Culpepper in *The English Physitians Enlarged* listed 369 medicines made of English herbs. He gives a complete method of physick:

"... Whereby a man may preserve his body in health or cure himself, being sick for three pence charge with such things only as grow in England, they being most fit for English herbs."

He teaches ways to make plasters, ointments, oils, syrups, etc. He is an astrologist and goes much by the stars. He tells when to gather herbs, how to dry them, and make useful compounds.

Even at the time he published this book he was trespassing on the monopoly claimed by recognized medical writers of his day. His works have been consecutively published down to our own day. The mainstream of medical writing was beginning to swerve off into the use of more and more chemicals.

Martin Lister (1638?-1712)

He was a zoologist, born in Yorkshire. He was the son of Martin Lister who was knighted in 1625. Lister was educated under an uncle, Sir Matthew Lister. He was made a fellow of the Royal Mandate in 1660.

He did a great deal of work on plants and spiders and was one of the earliest students on spiders. He wrote on meteorology, minerals, mollusos, medicine and antiquities.

He was a member of the Royal College of Physicians and in 1694 was chosen censor. Lister was appointed second physician in ordinary to Queen Ann. His fame was mostly in the field of zoology.

William Salmon (1644-1713)

He lived near the gates of St. Bartholomew's Hospital and obtained patients that could not be accepted.

Salmon was skilled in arts, engraving, etching, painting, furnishing, coloring, and dying.

He made a pill that sold for three shillings a box and was good for all diseases.

Peter Smith

His father, Hezekiah Smith of Jersey, was called Indian doctor.

Peter Smith wrote *Indian Doctor Dispensatory* in 1813 in which he said:

> *"Men seldom have wit enough to prize and take care of their health until they have lost it – and doctors often know not how to get their bread deservedly, until they have no teeth to chew it."*

Samuel Thomson (1769-1845)

Samuel Thomson was born February 9, 1969, to John and Hannah Thomson.

He developed the Thomsonian System and wrote 3 books: *A Brief Sketch of Cause and Treatment of Disease, Materia Medica and Family Physician, New Guide to Health or Botanic Family physician.*

He died October 4, 1845.

MISHNAH HERBAL REFERENCES

Some Mishnah references to herbs:

Amaranth – Shev 9:1
Fennel (asafetida) –Shab 20:3
                          Av-Zar 2:7
Balm – Shev 7:6
Barley – Kil 1:1
         Pres 2:5
Hyacinth Bean – Kil 1:1-1-2
                     Ma'as 4:7
Caraway – Kil 2-5
Carob – Pe'ah 1:5
Chicory – Shev 7:1
          Pres 2:6
          Kil 1-2
Citron – Ma'as 1:4 – 5:8
        Bik 2:6
Cress – Ma'as 4:5
Fenugreek – Kil 2:5
             Ter 10:5
Ginger – Shev 7:1, 2
Hyssop – Neg 14:6
           Par 11:7
Knobweed – Shab 14:3
Mint – Uk 1:2
Mulberry – Ma'as 1:2
Mustard – Kil 1:2; 1:5
Pepper – Shab 6:5
          Bezah 2:8
Safflower – Kil 2:8
            Uk – 3:5
            Shev 7:1
Saffron – Nid 2:6
Savory – Shev 8:1
          Ma'as 3:9
Sesame – Shev 2:7

Hal 1:4
Sorrel – Kil 1:3
Thyme – Shev 8:1; Ma'as 3:9

BIBLICAL REFERENCES

The Scriptures speak of herbs as if it were common knowledge.

In the beginning the Lord told Adam that fruit and herbs would be his meat, in Genesis 1:29 it states:

"And God said, behold, I have given you every herb bearing seed, which is upon the face of all the earth, and every tree, in the which is the fruit of a tree yielding seed; to you it shall be for meat."

Romans 14:2:

"For one believeth he may eat all things: another, who is weak, eateth herbs."

I Corinthians 3:17:

"If any man defile the temple of God him shall God destroy; for the temple of God is holy, which temple ye are."

Ezekiel 14:12:

"And by the River upon the bank thereof, on this side and on that side, shall grow all trees for meat, whose leaf shall not fade, neither shall the fruit thereof be consumed: it shall bring forth new fruit according to his months, because their waters they issued out of the sanctuary: and the fruit thereof shall be for meat, and the leaf thereof for medicine."

Psalm 104:14:

"He causeth the grass to grow for the cattle, and herb for the service of man: that he may bring forth food out of the earth."

II Kings 19:26:

"Therefore their inhabitants were of small power, they were dismayed and confounded; they were as the grass of the field, and as the green herb, as the grass on the house tops, and as corn boasted before it be grown up."

Psalm 37:2:

"For they shall soon be cut down like the grass, and wither as the green herb."

Jeremiah 12:4:

"How long shall the land mourn, and the herbs of every field wither, for the wickedness of them that dwell therein? the beasts are consumed, and the birds; because they said, He shall not see our last end."

Deuteronomy 11:10:

"For the land, whither that goest in to possess it, is not as the land of Egypt, from whence ye came out, where thou sowedst thy seed, and wateredst it with thy foot, as a garden of herbs."

II Kings 4:39:

"And one went out into the field to gather herbs, and found a wild v ine, and gathered thereof wild gourds his lap full, and came and shred them into the pot of pottage: for they knew them not."

ADDITIONAL READING

Nung, Shev (Emperor), *Pen Trao or Great Herbal,* Egypt, 1911. Emperor Shev Nung lived 3,000 B.C. The book remained in print 4,000 years. The latest printing was done in Egypt 1911.

The Golden Mere of Medicine Encyclopedia, 40 volumes. Includes massage and acupuncture.

The Edwin Smith Papyrus. Contains many interesting herbal uses. Even gives a description of how to set a dislocation of the jaw closely resembling the method we use today.

BIBLIOGRAPHY

Abercrombie, David. *A Moral Discourse of the Power of Interest.* London: Dorman Newman, 1691.

Allen, Benjamin. *The Natural History of the Chalybeat and Purging Waters of England.* London: S. Smith, 1699.

Andrus, Hyram L. *God, Man, and the Universe.* Salt Lake City: Bookcraft, 1968.

Arbuthnot, John. *Characters of Times.* n.p., n.d.

Arbuthnot, John. *Characters of Letters.* n.p., n.d.

Arbuthnot, John. *English Bells Letters from A.D. 9012 A.D. 1834* London: M .W. Dunne, 1901

Arbuthnot, John. *And Essay Concerning the Nature of Ailments* London: J. Tonson, 1731

Arbuthnot, John. *Trip to North Wales,* n.p., n.d.

Bank, Allen E. and Taylor, Renée. *Hunza Land.* Long Beach: Whitehorn Publishing Company, n.d.

Banyer, Henry. *Pharmacopoeia Pauperum.* London: T. Warner, 1728

Barton, Benjamin Smith. *Collections for an Essay Towards Materia Medica of the United States.* Philadelphia: Way and Groff, 1798.

Beckett, William. *New Discoveries Relating to the Cure of Cancer.* London: George Strahan, 1712.

Berlu, John Jacob. *Treasury of Drugs Unlocked.* London: S. Clarke, 1733.

Bernard, Raymond. *Herbal Elixirs of Life.* Molelumn, California: Health Research, n.d.

Bicaise, Honore. *Manuale Medicorum.* London: Thomas Toy croft, 1659.

Blackmore, Richard. *A Treatise of the Spleen and Vapours.* London: J. Pemberton, 1725.

Boerhaave, Hermann. *Academical Lectures on the Theory of Physick.* London, 1743.

Boerhaave, Hermann. *And Essay on the Virtue and Efficient Cause of Magnetical Cures.* London, 1743.

Boerhaave, Hermann. *Instructions in Physick.*London: W. R., 1714.

Boerhaave, Hermann. *International Symposium in Commemoration of the Tercentenary of Boerhaave's Birth.* Leydon: 1968

Boerhaave, Hermann. *Experiments Concerning Mercury.* London: J. Roberts, 1734.

Boerhaave, Hermann. *A Treatise on the Venereal Disease and its Cure.* London: T. Cox. 1729.

Borlase, Edmond. *Latham Spaw in Lancashire.* London: Robert Clavel, 1670.

Brandt, Johanna. *The Grape Cure.* Catherine's, Ontario: Provoker Press, n.d.

Brown, Phelps. *Complete Herbalist, People Their Own Physicians.* n.p.,n.d,

Burdon, Henry. *The Fountain of Health; or, A View of Nature.* London: Henry Burdon, 1734.

Cheyne, George. *The English Malady.* London: George Strahan, 1733

Christopher, Dr. *School of Natural Healing, 20 Lessons.* Dr. Christopher's manuscript. PO Box 352, Provo, UT

Cockburn, William. *And Account of the Nature, Causes, Symptoms, and Cure of Loosenesses.* London: T. Howlat, 1710.

Cockburn, William. *A Continuation of the Account of Nature...* London: T. Howlat 1697

Cockburn, William. *Sea Diseases.* London: George Strahan, 1715

Cockburn, William. *The Symptoms, Nature and Cure of Gonorrhea.* London: George Strahan, 1715.

Cocke, Thomas. *Kitchin Physick: Or Advice to the Poor.* London, J.B., 1675.

Cooley, Donald G. *Better Homes and Gardens Family Medical Guide,* New York: Meredith Press, 1966.

Cowper, William. *Myotomia Reformat.* London: Sam. Smith, 1694

Culpepper, Nicholas. *Complete Herbal.* Halifax: Milner and Sowerby, 1694.

Digby,, Kenelm, *A Discourse Concerning the Vegetation of Plants.* London: J.G., 1661.

Douglas, John. *A Syllabus of Chirurgical Operations.* London: J. Chandler, 1727.

Douglas, John. *A Short Dissertation of the Gout.* London: John Douglas, 1714.

Douglas, John. *A Short Account of Mortifications.* London: John Nourse, n.d.

Ehret, Arnold. *Mucusless Diet Healing System.* Beaumont, California: Ehret Publishing Company, n.d.

Francis, Dr. Samuel John. *Keys to Self-Understanding, Vol. III.* Santa Ana, California, n.d.

Gibby, J. Melvin. *Sand for the Rails.* Salt Lake City: Deseret Book Company, 1962

Groeneveldt, Jan. Lithologia. *A Treatise of the capstone and Gravel.* London: H.C., 1677.

Hartman, George. *The Family Physitian.* London: Richard Wellington, 1696.

Harvey, Gideon. *The Conclave of Physicians.* London: James Partridge, 1685.

Harvey, James. *Praesagium Medicum, or, The Prognostik Signs of Acute Diseases, n.p.,n.d.*

Helmont, Franciscus Mercurious van, 1618-1699. *The Paradoxal Discourse of... Concerning the Macrocosm and Microcosm.* London: J.C. and Freeman Collins, 1685.

Hortema, Hilton, *Man's Higher Consciousness,* Molelumn Hill, California: Health Research, n.d.

Hoxsey, Harry M. *You Don't Have to Die.* New York: Milestone Books, n.d.

Jackson, James Caleb. *How to Treat the Sick Without Medicine.* Dansville, New York: Austin, Jackson and Company, 1870.

Jacobson, Ruth. *Herbs of Utah.* (Manuscript) Provo, Utah.

Kloss, Jethro. *Back to Eden.* Longview publishing house, Tennessee, 1953.

LeClerc, Daniel. *The History of Physick.* London: D. Brown. 1699.

Lister, Martin. *Martin Lister Sex Exercitationes Medicinales.* London: S. Smith, 1694.

Livingston, Virginia Wuerthele-Caspe. *Cancer: A New Breakthrough.* Los Angeles: Nash Publishing Company, n.d.

Master Herbology, Ogden, Utah: Research Technical Service, n.d.

Meeks, Priddy. *Pretty Meeks Journal.*

*Merck's Manual.*Rahway, New Jersey: Merck, Sharp and Bohme Research Laboratories, n.d.

Meyer, Clarence. *The Herbalist*. Rand McNally and Company.

The Mishnah, oral teachings of Judaism. New York: Norton, 1970.

Newton, John. *Cosmographia, or a View of the Terrestrial and Coelestial Globes.* London: Thomas Passinger, 1679.

Pechey, John. *The London Dispensatory.* London: E. Collins. 1694.

Physicians' Desk Reference. 1973.

Prior, John A.; Silberstein, Jack S. *Physical Diagnosis.* St. Louis: The C.V. Mosby Company,n.d.

Rodman, Morton J.; Smith, Dorothy W. *Pharmacology and Drug Therapy in Nursing.* Philadelphia: J.B.Lippincott company, 1968.

Salmon, William. *Dr. Salmon's Last Legacy.* London: J.Dawks, n.d.

Doron Medicum. London: T. Dawks, 1683.

Family Dictionary. London: H. Rhodes, 1710.

Iatrica… The Practice of Curing Diseases. London: Nath Rolls 1694.

Paraleremata. London: George Conyers, 1689

Pharmacopoeia Londiniensis. London: J.Dawks, 1702.

Polygraphice: or The Arts of Drawing. London: Andrew Clark, 1675.

Paraxis Medica. London: J. B., 1707

Synopsis Medicinae. London: T. Dawks, 1679

Systemic Medicinale. London: T.Passinger, 1686.

Sawitz, William. *Medical Parasitology*. Toronto: New York Blankiston Company, n.d.

Shubert, Bruno H. *Survival of Mankind.* Molelumn Hill, California: Health Research.

Smith, Joseph. *The Dogmaticus or Family Physician,* n.p., 1829

Smith, Joseph, Jr. *Documentary History of the Church.* Salt Lake city: Deseret Book Company, 1948.

Smith, Peter. *Indian Doctor Dispensatory. n.p., n.d.*

Sweet, Muriel. *Common Edible and Useful Plants of the West.* Heraldsberg, California: Naturegraph Company, n.d.

Taber's Cyclopedia Medical Diet. Philadelphia: E. A. Davis Company, 1940.

Thomson, Samuel. *A Narrative of the Life of Medical Discoveries of Samuel Thomson.* Columbus, Ohio: Jarvis, Pike & Co. 1833.

Thomson, Samuel. *New Guide to Health or Botanic Family Physician. n.p., n.d.*

Tobe, John H. *Proven Herbal Remedies.* Canada: Provoker Press, n.d.

Tompkins, Peter; Bird, Christopher. *The Secret Life of Plants.* New York: Harper and Row, 1973.

Who Was Who in America, 1609-1896.

INDEX

Calcification - 30, 31
Calcium - 28, 30, 36, 38-40, 82, 88, 99, 170
Calluses - 79
Camels Hay - 212
Chamomile - 49, 50, 57, 62, 65, 78, 79, 82, 145, 147, 148, 154, 155, 158, 168, 169, 198, 211
Camphor - 211
Cancer - 29, 31-35, 39, 70, 75, 77, 82, 83, 84, 85, 86, 89, 114, 120, 122, 127, 128, 134, 140, 172, 195, 202, 208, 215
Canker Sores - 71, 78, 104, 123
Caraway - 50, 52, 212, 220
Carbuncles - 71, 77, 89, 109
Cardiac Herbs - 52
Carlyle, Thomas - 183
Carminative Herbs - 52
Carob - 149, 220
Carrageen - 62
Carrot - 55, 62
Cascara Sagrada - 60, 65, 79, 150, 167, 172
Castor Oil - 53, 121
Catalyst - 80, 93
Cataracts - 168
Catarrh - 37, 85, 86, 137, 193, 210
Cathartic Herbs - 52, 135, 164, 195
Catnip - 48, 50, 52, 54, 57, 61, 62, 79, 143, 145, 148, 151, 153, 157, 157, 168, 171
Cautery - 211
Cayenne - 36, 39, 43, 48, 62, 64, 80, 104, 105, 144, 147, 148, 152, 153, 154, 156, 157, 160, 165, 167-170, 195
Cedron - 81
Celandine - 46, 55, 57, 63, 81, 212
Celery - 30, 50, 56, 81, 155, 169
Centaury - 82, 167, 169, 170, 172
Cervi - 82
Chaparral - 29, 30, 34, 167
Chapped Hands - 148
Chemicals - 6, 15-17, 35, 36, 40, 43, 163
Chest - 128, 131, 134
Cheyne, George - 34

H

Peace - 174, 179, 180, 182-187
Peach - 50, 53, 56, 59, 60, 64, 100, 115, 148, 153, 155, 158, 159
Pechey, John; Purges For Eyes, Ears And Nose - 198
Pennyroyal - 115, 198
Peony - 38, 116, 125, 202, 209
Peppermint - 30, 50, 52, 65, 116, 150, 153, 155, 157, 159, 160, 168, 169, 171
Perfection - 181-182
Perfume - 131, 192
Peritonitis - 83, 8, 104
Periwinkle - 49, 51, 65, 117
Perspiration - 54, 76, 79, 80, 90, 94, 98, 115, 119, 124, 132, 134, 135, 139, 148, 149, 152, 155, 158
Peruvian Bark - 54, 59, 66, 118
Philosophy - 181, 215
Physicians - 161-163, 199
Piles: See Hemorrhoids
Pilewort - 51
Pinworms - 68, 121
Pink Root - 47, 66, 118, 143, 168
Pituitary Gland - 67
Plague - 68, 69, 81, 82, 84, 85, 90, 93, 100, 101, 103, 107, 110, 111, 116, 123, 126, 130, 133, 134, 138
Plantain - 46, 48, 49, 51, 53, 56, 118, 145, 150, 151, 157, 199, 212
Pleurisy - 47, 80, 104, 110, 119, 193, 202
Pleurisy Root - 49, 52, 55, 56, 57, 59, 119, 147, 154, 156, 160, 167
Pneumonia - 104, 105, 107, 125, 134,
Poison Bites - 68, 74, 81, 82, 93, 107, 124, 128, 138
Poison Ivy - 130
Poisoning - 43, 83, 88, 91, 124, 127
Poisons - 47, 76, 78, 201
Poke Root - 46, 53, 65, 119, 151, 154, 168, 170, 172
Pomegranate Peel - 199
Poplar - 59, 66, 120, 154
Poppy - 47
Potassium - 28, 30, 114, 170
Potato - 120, 143
Poultice - 71, 72, 79, 82, 83, 86, 89, 92, 98, 107, 111, 112, 114, 119, 130, 145, 147, 151, 158, 195, 211

Poultice Formula - 172
Power - 181-182
Pregnancy - 68, 98, 109, 115, 127, 131, 136
Preventative - 95
Preventative Medicine - 94, 95, 114
Prickly Ash - 46, 53, 61, 65, 120, 143, 144, 145, 159
Primrose - 63
Prostate - 76, 154
Prostate Formula - 172
Protein - 34
Psoriasis - 77, 85
Psyllium Seed - 53, 54, 61, 121, 149
Pulsatilla - 121, 143, 144
Pumpkin Seeds - 30, 34, 43, 56, 63, 66, 121, 172
Purgative Herbs - 63
Pus - 64, 88, 99, 199
Putrefaction - 48, 106, 121, 205, 208
Pyorrhea - 80, 96, 111, 156

Q
Quackery - 161, 202
Quaking Aspen - 120
Quassia - 47
Queen Of The Meadow - 51, 56, 122, 154, 158, 168
Quercetain - 122
Quinine - 44, 84, 125

R
Ragwort - 59
Raspberry Leaves – See Red Raspberry
Red Clover - 46, 54, 63, 122, 144, 149, 168
Red Raspberry - 46, 48, 63, 123, 147, 150, 160, 168
Red Root - 51, 59
Red Sage - 51, 55
Refrigerant Herbs - 64
Relaxant - 104, 105, 146, 148, 149, 151, 157, 159
Relaxation - 174, 176, 178
Religion - 181
Resolvent Herbs - 64

Syphilis - 73, 75, 77, 88, 89, 90, 103, 105, 114, 119, 120, 122, 126, 131, 140, 199
Systemic Lupus - 27

T
Tansy - 58, 66, 132, 147, 149, 151, 155, 172
Tapeworm - 121
Teeth - 50, 112
Testes - 83, 128
Testosterone - 127
Thomson, Samuel - 72, 79, 81, 94, 97, 105, 112, 121, 132, 139, 162, 164-166, 218
Thorn Apple - 47
Throat - 71, 83, 96, 103, 105, 110, 125, 127, 128, 134, 159, 160, 212
Thyme - 49, 52, 58, 132, 153, 169, 170, 198, 220
Thyroid - 119
Thyroid Formula - 172
Tobacco - 78
Tongue - 93, 121, 212
Tonic Herbs - 64, 65
Tonsils - 110, 159
Tooth Powder - 72
Toothache - 68, 69, 81, 85, 98, 107, 117, 121
Tormentils Root - 133
Trichinosis - 121
Tuber Bacillus -75
Tuberculosis - 77, 86, 90, 110, 113, 159
Tumors - 55, 64, 75, 83, 113, 139, 210
Turkey Corn - 56
Turpentine - 121, 211
Twin Leaf - 56
Twitching - 109
Twitching Eyelids - 88, 151
Typhoid Fever - 96, 111, 119, 139, 159

U
Ulcers -58, 72, 73, 75, 76, 80, 82, 83, 86, 87, 89, 97-99, 110, 112, 118, 119, 120, 121, 126, 129, 135, 137, 139, 159, 193, 199
Ulcer Formula -160

Wheezing - 134

White, Ellen; Herbs -17

White Ash - 48, 56, 60, 135

White Oak Bark - 48, 51, 146

White Pond Lily - 51, 53, 55

White Thorn Flowers - 212

White Willow - 51, 66, 135, 159

Whooping Cough - 67, 74, 75, 90, 95, 100, 104, 113, 115, 116, 122, 132, 135

Wild Alum Root - 48, 51,

Wild Carrot - 136,

Wild Lettuce - 46, 136, 171

Wild Oregon Grape - 46

Wild Turnip - 61

Wild Yam - 26, 30, 49, 136, 145, 167

Wilson's Disease - 41

Wintergreen - 48, 56, 58, 63, 66, 137, 146

Witch Hazel - 51

Witchcraft - 73

Womb - 109

Wood Betony - 30, 61, 137, 149, 151, 153, 155, 156, 159, 160, 171

Wood Sage -56, 66

Wood Sorrel - 138

Word of Wisdom - 166

Worms - 22, 47, 66, 67, 68, 70, 74, 76, 78, 80, 82, 88, 93, 99, 100, 101, 112, 115, 118, 120, 124, 124, 129, 132, 134, 138, 149

Wormwood - 37, 48, 50, 61, 138, 171, 198, 209, 211

Wounds - 54, 77, 79, 80, 82, 83, 86, 88, 89, 92, 96, 111, 112, 115, 118, 122, 125, 127, 137, 210

Y

Yarrow -46, 51, 55, 56, 63, 65, 66, 139, 147, 149, 150, 160, 167, 168, 169, 170, 172,

Yellow Dock -46, 51, 54, 63, 66, 80, 139, 144, 145, 161, 168, 171

Yellow Fever - 80, 161

Yellow Jaundice -110, 125, 139, 204

Yerba Santa - 59

Young, Brigham; Happiness - 189